Psychiatric Mental Health Psychopharmacology Project

AMERICAN NURSES ASSOCIATION

American Nurses Association
Task Force on Psychopharmacology
1992-1994

Michele T. Laraia, M.S.N., R.N.,Task Force Chair

Linda S. Beeber, Ph.D., R.N.

Gloria B. Callwood, Ph.D., R.N.

Susan Caverly, M.A., R.N.

Jeanne Anne Clement, Ed.D., R.N.

Faye Gary, Ed.D., R.N.

Norman L. Keltner, Ed.D., R.N.

Mary Ann Nihart, M.A., R.N.

Lawrence Scahill, M.S.N., M.P.H., R.N.

Susan Simmons-Alling, M.S.N., R.N.

Sarah R. Stanley, M.S., R.N., C.N.A., C.S.

Sandra Talley, M.N., R.N., A.N.P.

This project was completed with support from the Center for Mental Health Services (formerly NIMH), Division of Clinical Training Branch. Special thanks to project consultants and consumer panel:

Carol Bush, Ph.D., R.N.

Karen Soeken, Ph.D.

Winifred Carson, Esq.

Barbara Huff

Evelyn McElroy, Ph.D., R.N.

Vickie Cohn

ISBN 1-55810-104-7

Published by American Nurses Publishing
600 Maryland Avenue, SW
Suite 100 West
Washington, DC 20024-2571

PMH-13 10M 5/94

Table of Contents

Foreword

This publication is a summary of the work of the American Nurses Association Psychopharmacology Task Force and represents two years of activities, including the completion of the document.

In recent decades, the National Institute of Mental Health (NIMH) has supported the education and training of health care providers for the chronically mentally ill and their families. Psychiatric mental health nurses, from their biopsychosocial perspective, bring to the psychopharmacologic care of patients and families opportunities for medication teaching, administration, management, therapeutic maintenance, integration with the spectrum of interventions, and interdisciplinary collaboration with other health care providers. These established nursing functions are within the scope of psychiatric mental health nursing practice and are ones that are positively received by both patients and families. Care and caring have been and continue to be the cornerstone of nursing delivery of services.

The scientific advances of the past decade are changing the understanding of the human brain, mental illness, and biochemical treatments of mental disorders. Psychiatric nurses must continuously integrate the neurosciences, particularly psychopharmacology, into nursing practice to ensure safe and effective care of people with mental illness and the advancement of the specialty. To facilitate this ongoing process, the American Nurses Association (ANA) and NIMH funded the *Psychiatric Mental Health Nursing Psychopharmacology Project* in 1992.

Introduction

Michele T. Laraia, M.S.N., R.N.
Sarah R. Stanley, M.S., R.N., C.N.A., C.S.

The use of psychopharmacologic agents to treat mental illness has revolutionized the manner in which consumers of mental health services and the mental health professions view etiology, diagnosis, treatment, and cost of mental health care in this country. Consequently, there have been a number of important changes in the mental health field in recent decades.

For example, the national research agenda in mental health has been altered to promote evolving information and technologies. Mental health advocacy groups have been formed and have become a valuable voice in defining the mental health agenda today. The role of psychopharmacologic agents, both as research "probes"—unraveling the etiologies of mental illness and the bases of human behavior—and as powerful treatment tools, which may eventually reach every patient with psychiatric symptoms at one time or another, has expanded to levels of unprecedented sophistication in just a few brief decades.

In response, the roles of the four core mental health professions: psychiatric nursing, psychiatry, psychology, and social work, are being examined and refined to meet these new challenges. The multifaceted nature of mental illness and the complex care required for persons with mental illness necessitate the advantages afforded by the combined efforts of each discipline in the field of mental health care. Interdisciplinary collaboration will continue to provide the vehicle necessary for the most effective treatment and research efforts for the millions of persons suffering from these devastating illnesses.

In this, the "Decade of the Brain," the concerted attempts to apply neuroscientific principals to the understanding and treatment of mental illness will only become more pronounced. These efforts will result in new approaches to the diagnoses and treatments of mental illness, as well as elicit new hope for those who are consumers of mental health services. To best serve the needs of the many people with mental illness, and to remain effective health care providers and capable colleagues within the interdisciplinary mental health care arena, it is imperative that psychiatric mental health nurses remain actively involved in these rapid advances in the mental health field.

At this midpoint of the 90s, the specialty of psychiatric mental health nursing is at a critical juncture and should be prepared to move forward in the direction of future education, treatment, and research in the field of mental health. Meeting these challenges assures that patients and families will have access to the expert skills and resources of one of the largest groups of mental health care professionals, psychiatric nurses. At no other point in modern time has there been such a clearly defined window of opportunity for the specialty of psychiatric mental health nursing to advance in the science and art of mental health care.

Psychiatric nurses are among the primary health care professionals working on a daily basis with the long-term management of psychiatric patients on the continuum of prevention, diagnosis, treatment, maintenance, and rehabilitation. Given the present array of treatment options, this nursing management includes considerable attention to psychopharmacological agents, concurrent health problems, and complex interactions between behavioral, emotional, physiological, and psychopharmacologic events.

Psychiatric mental health nurses are unique in that their training and experience enable them to assess the biological as well as psychosocial needs of patients. Psychiatric mental health nurses will continue to refine and demonstrate their long-standing role in the mental health field, particularly regarding psychopharmacologic treatment and the education of patients and their families about psychopharmacologic agents. The American Nurses Association Psychopharmacology Project was conceptualized to evaluate and advance the scope of psychiatric nursing practice with respect to psychopharmacology and related neurosciences for both the psychiatric nurse clinician with a baccalaureate undergraduate nursing degree and the advanced-practice psychiatric clinical nurse specialist with a graduate degree in psychiatric mental health nursing.

Purpose

The purpose of the ANA Psychopharmacology Project is to improve psychopharmacologic treatment and educational services to persons with serious mental illness and their families by improving the expertise of psychiatric nurses to deliver those services.

Objectives

The specific objectives of the Psychopharmacology Project were:

1. to determine how well nursing education prepares nurses for practice in the treatment of the mentally ill with respect to psychopharmacology and related neurosciences;

2. to determine how nursing as a profession facilitates the continued expertise of psychiatric nurses with respect to the evolving content of psychopharmacology and related neurosciences;

3. to define the psychopharmacologic and neuroscientific knowledge base necessary in contemporary psychiatric nursing practice; and,

4. to develop guidelines for psychiatric mental health nurses in psychopharmacology and related neurosciences for the treatment of persons with mental illness.

Methods

The Psychopharmacology Project used several methods to achieve these objectives:

ANA appointed a representative group of psychiatric mental health nurses to the Psychopharmacology Task Force. These 12 psychiatric mental health nurse specialists are recognized for their interest, expertise, and leadership in psychopharmacologic treatment, education, and research. The task force membership reflects a diversity in gender, race, age, affiliation, educational background, state nurses associations (SNAs), and specialty organizations. Task Force members assumed primary responsibility for meeting the objectives of the Psychopharmacology Project. The members of the Psychopharmacology Task Force and their affiliations are listed at the beginning of this book and in Appendix 1.

Five *content* areas were defined by the task force to be used as guidelines for organizing the information gathered during the Psychopharmacology Project. These content areas were selected from literature reviews as well as the collective expertise of the task force members regarding the scope of practice of psychiatric mental health nurses working with psychopharmacologic agents.

The task force members met to plan the implementation of the Psychopharmacology Project and to identify relevant issues in psychopharmacology in nursing practice. This long list of issues was then organized into the following five content areas:

- Neurosciences
- Psychopharmacology
- Assessment
- Clinical Management
- Legal/Ethical Issues

Evaluation of the nursing environment was completed. The nursing *environment* is defined as the contribution of the nursing profession regarding education, publications, presentations, and practice in psychiatric nursing. It is from this environment that psychiatric mental health nurses learn about and remain current in psychopharmacology. The environment was evaluated in several ways:

Education: An *educational survey* was developed and sent to every nursing program accredited by the National League for Nursing (NLN). Schools of nursing were asked to provide detailed information about their curricula on psychiatric nursing, psychopharmacology, and related neurosciences.

Publications and Presentations: The following resources were reviewed for content in psychopharmacology and related neurosciences:

- psychiatric nursing textbooks,
- psychiatric nursing journals,
- computer resources and videos, and
- psychiatric nursing conference programs.

Practice: A *National Psychopharmacology Working Conference* of psychiatric mental health nurses recommended by their SNAs was convened. The purpose of this conference was to determine nurses use of psychopharmacological interventions in their work with mentally ill patients and their families, and the psychopharmacologic and neuroscientific content that psychiatric nurses in practice need to know.

Consumers of mental health services were invited to participate in the Psychopharmacology Project. Representatives of the National Alliance for the Mentally Ill and The Federation of Families for Children's Mental Health attended the National Psychopharmacology Working Conference and shared their perspectives with the conference participants.

The Psychopharmacology Task Force synthesized the information gained from the Psychopharmacology Project methods described above and developed the *Psychopharmacology Guidelines for Psychiatric Mental Health Nurses*. This document presents guidelines for psychiatric mental health nurses to work at optimal proficiency with patients who receive psychopharmacologic agents as treatments for mental illness. The guidelines are presented in full in Part II, Section 5.

PART I

The Psychiatric Mental Health Nursing Environment for Psychopharmacology and Related Neurosciences

Education Survey

Lawrence Scahill, R.N., M.S.N., M.P.H.
Michele T. Laraia, R.N., M.S.N.

The Education Survey was sent to all schools of nursing in the United States accredited by the National League for Nursing (NLN) as of October 1992. The purpose of the survey was to determine psychopharmacology and neuroscience content of curricula of nursing programs at the undergraduate and graduate (master's) levels.

Methods

To define the content and scope of the Education Survey during its development, the task force explored specific subject areas from which the survey questions were fashioned. Separate versions of the survey were developed for undergraduate and graduate programs. However, a core group of questions was included in both versions to permit comparisons across educational levels. The questions were then given to a statistician-consultant who developed the format for the questionnaire.

The surveys were sent to 240 graduate programs and 1,498 undergraduate programs throughout the country in the fall of 1992. The surveys were sent to the dean of each school with a cover letter (Appendix 2) that explained the purpose of the survey and requested that the survey be referred to the most appropriate faculty member for completion. No reminders or repeat mailings were sent. A 10 percent random sample of the non-respondents was contacted by telephone, permitting some examination of the non-participants. Of the 1,738 surveys mailed, 881 were returned (Table 1).

There were no significant differences in the rate of response by region for either the graduate or undergraduate programs (Table 2), nor were there any differences

TABLE 1

Response Rate

	TOTAL SENT	TOTAL RETURNED	PERCENT RETURNED
Graduate programs	240	143	59.6%
Undergraduate programs	1498	738	49.3%
TOTALS	1738	881	50.7%

TABLE 2

Undergraduate and Graduate Response Rate by Region

South	49%
Midwest	47%
North Atlantic	51%
West	47%

in the response rates for the three types of undergraduate programs (Table 3).

TABLE 3
The Educational Survey: Undergraduate Response Rate by Type of Program

Baccalaureate	49%
Associate Degree	45%
Diploma	53%

Results

UNDERGRADUATE

The sample of undergraduate schools that returned the survey is described in Table 4. Of the total of 738 responding undergraduate schools, 79 percent ($n = 583$) included a specific psychiatric nursing course in their curriculum. This figure was fairly consistent across program types (Table 5).

TABLE 4
Surveys Returned by Undergraduate Programs

PROGRAM	NUMBER RETURNED	PERCENT OF THE TOTAL SAMPLE
Baccalaureate (B.S./N.)	248	33.6%
Associate Degree (A.D.)	377	51.1%
Diploma Programs	77	10.4%
Two-Degree Programs	36	4.9%

Note: $N = 738$.

TABLE 5
Undergraduate Programs with a Specific Psychiatric Nursing Course

B.S./N.	83%
A.D.	76%
Diploma	78%

Although a majority of the responding schools included a specific course for psychiatric nursing, only a small minority included more than one course. On average, this single course consisted of 36 hours of classroom instruction and 90 hours of clinical practicum.

Programs that do not have a specific psychiatric nursing course (21 percent) reported that approximately 15 percent of the total curriculum covers psychiatric nursing, curriculum varied from 1 percent to 35 percent. For 17 percent of the programs with an integrated curriculum, the psychiatric nursing content represents less than 10 percent of the total curriculum and for 13 percent of the programs, the content represents between 21 percent and 35 percent.

Virtually all programs, whether they had a specific course in psychiatric nursing or not, included some clinical experience in a psychiatric setting. This experience was almost exclusively inpatient.

These undergraduate programs have an average of 60 graduates per year and have approximately 2.3 full-time faculty in psychiatric nursing. Most of these programs reported having faculty members with a master's degree in psychiatric nursing, though only 20 percent of the responding schools have a doctorally prepared faculty member for psychiatric nursing.

Course Content: Though most programs teach all treatment modalities, the two primary treatment modalities covered in the undergraduate programs are individual therapy and milieu therapy. These approaches were taught in over 95 percent of the programs and were considered the primary modalities by at least half of the programs. By contrast, just over one-third reported that somatic therapies were presented as primary. Table 6 reports curriculum content for undergraduate schools.

TABLE 6
Psychiatric Nursing Curriculum for Undergraduate Schools

CONTENT	N	%
Specific course in psychiatric nursing[1]	583	78.9
Individual therapy as primary treatment modality	531	71.9
Milieu therapy as primary treatment modality	369	50.0
Somatic therapies as primary treatment modalities	287	38.8

Note: $N = 738$.
[1] Programs without a specific course in psychiatric nursing provided relevant content in an "integrated curriculum."

Nearly all the programs reported that their curricula included course content (either required or available as optional) on the divisions of the central nervous system (94 percent), functional organization of the brain (93 percent), mechanisms of neurotransmission (96 percent), and biological theories of psychiatric illness (98 percent). Fewer have content concerning the relationship of endocrinology to behavior and mood (74 percent), or neuro-imaging (43 percent).

Survey results suggest considerable variability in the amount of time spent on these topics (1.6 to 5.7 hours). Thus, it was not possible to ascertain from the survey how comprehensively these topics are covered.

Biological theories of mental illness and neuro-imaging tend to be taught in nursing departments by nurses whereas divisions of the central nervous system and functional organization of the brain tend to be taught outside the nursing department by persons other than nurses.

Regarding clinical psychopharmacology, over 90 percent of undergraduate program respondents reported they teach management of side effects, medication tolerance/dependence, identification of target symptoms, the importance of physical assessment and medical illness, medication interactions and long-term monitoring, and treating the elderly.

Approximately 60 percent of programs teach about the impact of race, gender, age, family history, and the use of behavioral rating scales on medication choice or management, though over half of the respondents acknowledged that these issues deserved more attention in their curricula.

Undergraduate nursing students are taught that nurses have responsibility for medication monitoring, teaching, documenting, and managing side effects, and physicians have the responsibility for decision making, selecting, prescribing, and discontinuing medication. While fewer than half of the programs teach the importance of collaboration with the patient and his or her family in selecting, managing, discontinuing, or documenting medication, just over 60 percent of programs teach collaboration with patient and family in monitoring medication.

Clinical Experience: Most undergraduate students provide direct care to a culturally and racially diverse patient population in public inpatient facilities. The clinical experience includes patient evaluation and participation in treatment planning. Undergraduate students are also involved in client education about medication, but only a small fraction of students administer medications in these clinical settings.

GRADUATE SCHOOLS

Of the 143 graduate nursing programs that returned questionnaires (from the original pool of 240) 80 (56

percent) did not have a specialty program for psychiatric nursing. The random 10 percent sample of non-respondents suggested that they were less likely to have a psychiatric nursing graduate program. Thus, the results presented here reflect the responses of the 63 programs that completed the survey and have a graduate program in psychiatric nursing. The largest number of graduate psychiatric nursing programs in this sample are found in the south, while the fewest are in the west (Table 7).

TABLE 7
Geographic Distribution of Graduate Psychiatric Nursing Program Respondents

REGION	NUMBER
South	25 (40%)
Midwest	16 (26%)
North Atlantic	12 (19%)
West	9 (15%)
TOTAL	62

Note: N = 63. One response for "region" was missing.

The 63 master's psychiatric nursing programs graduate approximately 441 students per year (mean = 7). In response to questions about treatment modalities taught, 61 percent of the programs answered individual, 59 percent group, and 58 percent family. Approximately one-third of the programs teach somatic treatments and milieu. When asked about the *primary* treatment modality taught, 81 percent reported individual, followed by 56 percent group and 45 percent family.

Course content: A majority of the graduate programs (41/63) required at least some psychopharmacology content in their curricula (Table 8). Less than one-fourth of the graduate programs (n = 14) offered psychopharmacology as an option and four programs neither required nor offered psychopharmacology (responses on

TABLE 8
Psychopharmacology in Graduate Psychiatric Nursing Programs

PSYCHOPHARMACOLOGY INSTRUCTION	N	%
Required	41	65.1
Optional	14	22.2
Unavailable	4	6.3
Missing data	4	6.3
Offered through a specific course	8	12.7

Note: N = 63.

this item by the remaining four programs were incomplete and could not be assessed). Although a majority reported that psychopharmacology was included in their curricula, only eight programs offered a specific course for psychopharmacology. Lecture hours ranged from one to a full course of 18 hours (Table 9).

TABLE 9

Frequency Distribution for Number of Lecture Hours for Psychopharmacology Content Graduate Programs

HOURS	PROGRAMS
1-3	10 (31.3%)
4-6	4 (12.5%)
7-6	3 (9.4%)
10-12	6 (18.8%)
13-15	1 (3.1%)
16-18	1 (3.1%)
18	7 (21.9%)

Note: Of the 56 programs offering this content, only 32 responded to this item.

Psychopharmacology content tends to be offered within the nursing department (91 percent of the programs), or in collaboration with another discipline (9 percent). Psychopharmacology content tends to be organized by both medication classification and psychiatric disorder (60 percent of the programs), rather than only by one or the other. Lecture (89 percent of the programs) and discussion (84 percent of the programs) are the predominant methods of instruction.

Based on survey responses, specific deficiencies were implied in areas such as the impact of gender and family history on drug selection, psychopharmacologic treatment considerations for children, research strategies in clinical psychopharmacology, and the use of standardized rating scales.

Over one-half of the respondents (38/63) reported that psychiatric nursing course work emphasized psychodynamic, interpersonal, and psychosocial causes of mental illness. By contrast, only a small minority of programs include course content on biological and genetic etiologies (4/63).

Furthermore, the amount of neurobiology presented in graduate school curricula appears to be limited. Ten to fifteen percent do not offer content on the structure and function of the brain or the relationship of endocrinology to behavior and mood. Where neuroscience content is taught, it tends to be taught within the nursing department, with an average of less than three lecture hours. These results are consistent with the relatively low percentage of programs offering content on the biological etiology of mental illness.

Topics least likely to be included are those psychopharmacology content areas dealing with special populations, especially among programs in the south as compared to those in the west. Content about research strategies in psychopharmacology and the use of standardized behavioral rating scales are included in approximately one-half of the programs with psychopharmacology content.

In virtually all of the 63 graduate programs, students were taught that there is a high level of nursing responsibility in clinical management (monitoring, teaching, and documenting and managing side effects) compared to that for physicians and pharmacists. This same level of responsibility is not apparent in clinical decision making (securing informed consent, choosing medication, discontinuing medication, and prescribing medication)—all of which are relegated to physicians.

Despite the growing number of states that have granted prescriptive authority to advanced practice nurses, only one-third of the programs teach their graduate students that advanced practice nurses can prescribe medication.

Clinical Experience: In 58 of the 63 programs (92 percent), graduate students are providing direct care in public outpatient facilities to a racially and culturally diverse patient population. Table 10 shows the focus of direct care responsibility for graduate students in clinical training. In keeping with the outpatient settings,

---

TABLE 10

Clinical Care Experience in Psychiatric Nursing Graduate Programs

CLINICAL SERVICE	PERCENTAGE OF STUDENTS	
	>50%	<50%
Assessment	93	7
Treatment, planning, evaluation	90	10
Individual psychotherapy	89	12
Patient education	61	39
Monitoring treatment	60	40
Family education	31	69
Administration of		
Nonpsychopharmacologic medication	10	90
Psychopharmacologic medication	18	83

Note: Percentages may not add to 100 due to rounding.
N = 63.

graduate students in these psychiatric nursing programs are not administering medication.

Most programs acknowledged the importance of concurrent physical illness, physical assessment, identification of target symptoms, and medication interaction in the choice of pharmacologic agent. However, the extent to which these assessment skills are included in graduate programs could not be ascertained from this survey.

COMPARISONS ACROSS PROGRAMS

One possible interpretation of the relative absence of content in psychopharmacology and related neurosciences in graduate programs is that schools assume these areas were covered in undergraduate programs. To evaluate this possibility, selected items were compared across undergraduate and graduate programs.

Direct Care Experiences: The proportion of programs reporting that most students have responsibility for treatment planning/evaluation, family education, and administration of medications is lowest for associate degree and highest for master's. Responsibility for patient education and assessment is highest in the B.S./N. programs (Table 11).

Psychiatric Nursing Content: Typically, a lower proportion of master's programs included specific psychi-

atric nursing content areas included in the survey when compared to B.S./N. and A.D. programs, with the exception of the advisability of malpractice insurance (Table 12).

TABLE 12

Psychiatric Nursing Content across Programs

CONTENT	A.D. %	B.S./N. %	MASTER'S %
Patient's right to refuse medication	99	100	94
Confidentiality re: psychopharmacologic agents	94	91	83
Risk/benefit ratio in psychopharmacologic Rx	96	96	86
Administration of psychopharmacologic agents against patient's will	97	96	82
Involuntary and voluntary treatment	99	100	90
Clinical decision-making regarding PRN psychopharmacologic agents	92	89	77
Psychopharmacologic agents as chemical restraint	93	95	85
Alternatives to psychopharmacologic treatment	99	99	90
Documentation related to psychopharmacologic treatment	92	96	77
Advisability of malpractice insurance in psychiatric settings	70	76	87

TABLE 11

Direct Care Experiences Comparison across Programs

CLINICAL SERVICE	PERCENT OF STUDENTS	A.D. %	B.S./N. %	MASTER'S %
Assessment	<75%	23	15	23
	>75%	77	85	77
Treatment planning/ evaluation	<75%	48	33	21
	>75%	52	67	79
Family education about pharmacologic treatment	<75%	68	59	29
	>75%	32	41	71
Patient education about pharmacologic treatment	<75%	62	45	57
	>75%	38	55	43
Administration of non-psychopharmacologic medications	none	64	51	42
	some	36	49	58
Administration of psychopharmacologic medications	none	62	49	50
	some	38	51	60

Psychopharmacologic Content: Fewer differences were noted concerning psychopharmacologic content in the curricula, with differences emerging for only eight of the 19 content areas queried (Table 13).

Neuroscience Content: A significantly lower percentage of master's programs, as compared to A.D. or B.S./N. programs, require neuroscience content. While over 90 percent of the A.D. and B.S./N. programs require content about the central nervous system, organization of the brain, neurotransmission, biological bases of mental illness, and psychopharmacology, fewer than 70 percent of the master's programs require this content. Percentages are lower for endocrinology related to mood and behavior, but the same pattern is evident (Table 14). Where content is available, it tends to be offered in the nursing department for master's students, and outside nursing for undergraduate students.

TABLE 13

Areas of Significant Differences across Programs for Psychopharmacology Content

CONTENT	A.D. %	B.S./N. %	MASTER'S %
Impact of family history on drug selection	56	63	73
Impact of gender on drug selection	46	50	73
Importance of physical assessment prior to drug selection	99	98	93
Detoxification	93	92	74
Extrapyramidal symptoms	100	100	96
Management of drug side effects	100	100	93
Use of standardized behavioral rating scales	41	48	61
Tardive dyskinesia	100	100	96

TABLE 14

Percent of Programs Requiring Neuroscience Content

CONTENT	A.D. %	B.S./N. %	MASTER'S %
Divisions of the central nervous system	95	95	57
Functional organization of the brain	93	94	53
Mechanisms of neurotransmission	95	94	63
Endocrinology related to behavior and mood	77	84	53
Biological theories of mental illness	94	96	78
Neuro-imaging	40	44	39 ns
Psychopharmacology	97	97	69

ns = differences across programs are not significant.

Discussion

This report provides preliminary results of a 28-item survey sent to undergraduate and graduate schools of nursing accredited by the NLN as of October 1992. Although there was no evidence that the non-respondents were markedly different from respondents, the rate of non-participation makes it difficult to generalize from the survey. Therefore, the findings should be viewed with caution.

Nonetheless, certain trends emerge from the survey for both undergraduate and graduate curricula that war-rant further discussion. In undergraduate programs nursing students apparently receive an overview of etiological theories of mental illness, but psychodynamic and psychosocial determinants are considered primary. This emphasis is juxtaposed with the revolution that is occurring in the scientific community concerning the biological underpinnings for the major mental illnesses. Moreover, the pace of research in the neurosciences is accelerating at an unprecedented rate and is having an almost daily impact on the field of mental health.

Graduate programs in psychiatric nursing appear to be preparing students to provide individual psychotherapy in outpatient settings. This emphasis may be out of step with the trend toward interdisciplinary and multi-modal treatment. Graduate programs seem to emphasize a high degree of responsibility for monitoring medications, but limited authority concerning the selection and discontinuation of medication. This trend was strongly evident in the survey, despite the growing number of states that have prescriptive authority for advanced practice nurses, and despite the growing debate in the health care industry regarding access, treatment, and reimbursement.

The findings from the survey suggest that nursing education be refined and rejuvenated to include up-to-date information in psychopharmacology and related neurosciences. Failure to do so will leave nurses unprepared for work in mental health as generalists and out of step as specialists.

To maintain professional respect from other nursing specialties, as well as health care colleagues from other disciplines and consumer advocates, psychiatric nursing cannot afford to withdraw from the challenge of contemporary mental health care. Psychiatric mental health nurses depend on the educational system for a solid base in the specialty from which they can continue to develop throughout their careers.

The specialty is dependent upon the educational system to attract students to psychiatric nursing. The educational system sets the tone for the future of nursing, and determines the growth, skills, contributions, and success of the specialty of psychiatric mental health nursing. Thus, nursing education is in the position to make a major contribution to the advancement of the specialty of psychiatric mental health nursing in the fields of psychopharmacology and related neurosciences.

Publications and Resources

The environmental assessment also included a comprehensive review of current textbooks, journal articles, computer resources/videos, and conferences specifically targeting psychiatric mental health nurses. This effort was undertaken to determine whether these resources are providing comprehensive and ongoing information to enable psychiatric mental health nurses to remain current with the state of the art and science of psychopharmacology and related neurosciences.

These four categories of publications and resources were selected because they represent sources of knowledge that would include information across a continuum of time. For example, conferences could be expected to represent the most up-to-date material, and to be the most responsive to nursing consumer demand, followed by journal articles and computer programs.

Textbooks would be the most likely to offer a structuring of existing knowledge into more comprehensive models and would serve as landmarks by which advancement of the specialty could be judged. In keeping with the fast pace with which knowledge in these fields is growing, one would also expect that a continuum of increasing information in psychopharmacology and related neurosciences would be evident over time.

This summary will review the process of data collection for each of the respective areas and highlight the neurobiological and psychopharmacological knowledge noted therein.

Textbooks

Sandra Talley, M.N., R.N., A.N.P.

The most recent editions of available psychiatric nursing textbooks providing a comprehensive review of the specialty were selected for this review (Table 15). A total of 12 texts were reviewed. Texts with a specific, narrow focus, such as crisis intervention or assessment, were not included. Any portions of the texts (e.g., chapters, parts of chapters, appendices, and tables) covering psychopharmacology and related neurosciences also were reviewed.

TABLE 15
Psychiatric Nursing Textbooks Reviewed
Birckhead *Psychiatric Mental Health Nursing*, 1989
Burgess *Psychiatric Nursing*, 5th Ed., 1990
Cook and Fontaine *Essentials of Mental Health Nursing*, 1991
Gary and Kavanagh *Psychiatric Mental Health Nursing*, 1991
Haber, McMahon, Price-Hoskins, Sideleau *Comprehensive Psychiatric Nursing*, 4th Ed., 1992
Janosik and Davies *Psychiatric Mental Health Nursing*, 2nd Ed., 1992
Keltner, Schwecke, Bostron *Psychiatric Nursing: A Psychotherapeutic Management Approach*, 1991
Murray and Huelskoetter *Psychiatric Mental Health Nursing*, 3rd Ed., 1991
McFarland and Thomas *Psychiatric Mental Health Nursing*, 1991
Stuart and Sundeen *Principles and Practice of Psychiatric Nursing*, 4th Ed., 1991
Varacolis *Foundation of Psychiatric Mental Health Nursing*, 1990
Wilson and Kneisl *Psychiatric Nursing*, 4th Ed., 1992

The following questions were asked in the evaluation of texts for:

Psychopharmacological content: Were traditional as well as newer psychopharmacologic agents presented? Was there an integration of psychopharmacologic interventions with discussion of psychiatric disorders? How extensive was the content with respect to target symptoms, side effects, adverse reactions, drug interactions, nursing management, and patient education? Was there a consistent level of depth for all drug categories?

Related neuroscience content: How detailed and up-to-date were the biological theories of mental illness? Were sections on neuro-anatomy and neurophysiology included? Was there an integration of biological theory with behavior and psychopharmacological intervention? What background knowledge was provided to help the reader comprehend biological theories and interventions?

Each text was then rated for specific categories with the following scale:

3 = most comprehensive coverage
2 = comprehensive
1 = minimal coverage

The results of this assessment are presented in Table 16.

Summary

In general, there has been an increased attempt over time, given the publication dates of the texts, to present neurobiological and psychopharmacological content in a more up-to-date and sophisticated manner. Few authors presented a "most comprehensive coverage" of neurosciences related to mental illness, and many of the newer psychopharmacologic treatments were only "minimally covered." Several of the texts used illustrations and tables which greatly enhanced the presentation of this complex material.

TABLE 16

Nursing Environment Report Textbook Review

TEXTBOOKS	TRADITIONAL PSYCHOTROPIC DRUGS	COVERAGE OF NEWER PSYCHOPHARMACOLOGICAL AGENTS	COVERAGE OF SIDE EFFECTS UNTOWARD EFFECTS DRUG INTERACTIONS	BIOLOGICAL THEORIES OF MENTAL ILLNESS
Comprehensive Psychiatric Nursing, 4th ed., Haber, McMahon, Price-Hoskins, Sideleau, 1992	Chapter 2.5	Clozaril Prozac Tegretol Verapamil Valproic acid	Side effects; untoward effects; drug interactions 2.5	Biological theories 2.0
Essentials of Mental Health Nursing, Cook and Fontaine, 1991	Chapter 1.0	Prozac	Side effects; untoward effects 1.5	Neurotransmitters; brain imaging 1.0
Foundations of Psychiatric Mental Health Nursing, Varcarolis, 1990	Integrated appendix 1.5	Tegretol Prozac Valproic acid	Side effects; untoward effects 2.0	Biological theories 1.5
Principles and Practice of Psychiatric Nursing, 4th ed., Stuart and Sundeen, 1991	Chapter 2.5	Prozac Tegretol Valproic Acid Clozaril	Side effects; drug interactions; untoward effects 2.5	Brain imaging; neurotransmitters 1.5
Psychiatric Mental Health Nursing, Birckhead, 1989	Appendix integrated 1.5	Prozac	Side effects; untoward effects; drug interactions 1.5	1.0
Psychiatric Mental Health Nursing, Gary and Kavanagh, 1991	Integrated 2.0	Clozaril Tegretol Prozac	Side effects; untoward effects 2.0	Integrated content 2.0
Psychiatric Mental Health Nursing, 2nd ed., Janasik and Davies, 1989	Appendix integrated 2.5	Prozac Tegretol	Side effects; drug interactions; untoward effects 2.5	Biological theories 1.5

TABLE 16				

Nursing Environment Report Textbook Review (continued)

TEXTBOOKS	TRADITIONAL PSYCHOTROPIC DRUGS	COVERAGE OF NEWER PSYCHOPHARMACOLOGICAL AGENTS	COVERAGE OF SIDE EFFECTS UNTOWARD EFFECTS DRUG INTERACTIONS	BIOLOGICAL THEORIES OF MENTAL ILLNESS
Psychiatric Mental Health Nursing, 3rd ed., Murray and Huelskoetter, 1992	Integrated 1.0	Clozaril Tegretol	Side effects 1.5	Biological theories; some brain imaging 1.5
Psychiatric Nursing, 5th ed., Burgess, 1990	Chapter 2.5	Tegretol Valproic Acid Clozaril	Side effects; drug interactions; untoward effects 2.5	Biological theories 1.5
Psychiatric Nursing, 4th ed., Wilson and Kniesl, 1992	Chapter; appendix 2.5	Prozac Tegretol Clozaril	Side effects; untoward effects 2.0	Neuro-anatomy; biological theories; neurotransmitters 3
Psychiatric Mental Health Nursing, McFarland and Thomas, 1991	Chapter 2.0	Clozaril Prozac Tegretol	Side effects; untoward effects 2.0	Neurotransmitters; brain imaging 2.0
Psychiatric Nursing: A Psychotherapeutic Management Approach, Keltner, Schwecke, Bostron, 1991	Separate chapters and integrated 2.5	Prozac Tegretol Clozaril	Side effects; untoward effects; drug interactions 2.5	Biological theories; neurotransmitters; brain imaging; neurophysiology 2.5

Note: 3 = most comprehensive coverage, 2 = comprehensive coverage, 1 = minimal coverage.

Journals

Michele T. Laraia, R.N., M.S.N.

The National Library of Medicine (NLM) was contacted for a listing of all psychiatric mental health nursing journals. There are seven currently being published worldwide, and all seven are in the English language. Five are published in the United States, one in Australia, and one in Canada. Ten additional psychiatric mental health nursing journals are listed as "closed," no longer published—seven English-language, and three non-English language.

A five-year (1988-1992) computer search utilizing the Comprehensive Index of Nursing and Allied Health Literature (CINAHL) was conducted using the following key words: psychopharmacology and biological psychiatry. The CINAHL database was selected because it searches the nursing as well as the allied health literature, and because many of the other health care databases, such as MedLine, do not include many of the nursing journals. CINAHL is, therefore, the database most commonly used by nursing students as well as nurses in practice, education, and research for computerized literature reviews of nursing journal publications.

Findings

The CINAHL search resulted in the retrieval of three articles from the five United States psychiatric nursing journals on the topics of psychopharmacology and biological psychiatry. Forty-eight articles using these two key words were retrieved for the same time span from nursing journals of specialties other than psychiatric nursing. A manual search was then conducted of the five United States psychiatric nursing journals for 1988 to 1992. Each article was scanned for relevant content, regardless of the title or the abstract.

This investigation revealed that the content of many articles in psychiatric nursing journals reviewed was not necessarily reflected in the title or the abstract, making a key-word-generated electronic database search for psychopharmacology and biological psychiatry unproductive. Seventy articles including relevant psychopharmacology and biological psychiatry content were found in the manual search of the same psychiatric nursing journals originally included in the electronic CINAHL search. The number of articles with psychopharmacologic or neurobiologic content are listed by journal (Table 17) and topics (Table 18).

TABLE 17				
Biological/Psychopharmacological Articles by Journal				
JOURNAL	*PSYCHOBIOLOGY*	*SPECIFIC DISORDER*	*PSYCHOPHARMACOLOGY*	*TOTAL*
Archives of Psychiatric Nursing	9	4	5	18
1992 7 1989 2				
1991 4 1988 1				
1990 4				
Journal of Psychosocial Nursing	2	4	21	27
1992 4 1989 3				
1991 8 1988 3				
1990 9				
Issues in Mental Health Nursing	0	2	3	5
1992 2 1989 0				
1991 0 1988 2				
1990 1				
Perspectives in Psychiatric Care	1	1	8	10
1992 2				
1991 4				
1990 4				
Journal of Child and Adolescent Psychiatric Nursing	3	5	2	10
1992 1 1990 5				
1991 2 1989 2				
GRAND TOTAL	*1988*	*1989*	*1990*	*1991*	*1992*
70	6	7	23	18	16

TABLE 18	
Summary of Articles on Psychopharmacology and Related Neurosciences Topics	
Imaging	1
Autism	1
Bipolar Disorder	1
Depression	1
Circadian Rhythms	1
Conduct Disorder	1
Panic Disorder	1
Genetics	2
Aggression	1
Anorexia	1
Bulimia	1
Developmental	1
Culture	1
Prozac	1
Carbamazepine	1
Carbamazepine/Valproate	1
Post-Traumatic Stress Disorder	1
Prescriptive Authority	2
Obsessive-Compulsive Disorder	2
Seasonal Affective Disorder	3
Tourette's Syndrome	1
Clozapine	4
Psychobiology	5
Schizophrenia	6
General Pharmacology (Side Effects, Nutrition, Patient Education, Role, Right to Refuse Medication, etc.)	27

Summary

These data suggest that the conventions for assigning key words regarding psychopharmacology and related neurosciences for psychiatric nursing journal searches may need to be re-evaluated. The difficulty in electronically searching the nursing literature for neuroscientific information is a distinct disadvantage to psychiatric nursing because it poses a barrier to the use of computer-generated databases for retrieval of relevant articles in specialty journals.

In addition, as the data from the manual search show, there is no comprehensive coverage of the fields of psychopharmacology and related neurosciences represented in the specialty journals targeting psychiatric mental health nurses. As evidenced in Table 18, there are many topics in psychopharmacology and related neurosciences relevant to psychiatric nurses that are not addressed in the five specialty journals reviewed.

Thus, it is important that the authors of psychiatric mental health nursing journal articles, as well as the publishers of these journals, increase focus in the future on the key word concept of topic identification for computer-generated database searches, as well as increase the coverage of psychopharmacology and the neurosciences in a comprehensive manner.

From the NLM information, it appears that journals which focus specifically on topics relevant to psychiatric mental health nursing are few in number, and have a history of not remaining viable. There are few specialty journals in psychiatric mental health nursing, with few articles relevant to psychopharmacology and related neurosciences, and they are very difficult to access electronically. The psychiatric nurse who wants to be up-to-date in these important fields must access the journals of other health specialties and disciplines as well as psychiatric mental health nursing journals.

Computer Resources and Videos

Linda S. Beeber, Ph.D., R.N.

A search for computer resources and videos was conducted utilizing the following sources:

- Direct communication with the Association of Educational Communication and Technology and the Fuld Institute for Technology in Nursing Education.
- On-Line computer resource networks.
- Review of 1992-1993 catalogues for computer-assisted learning materials.
- Direct communication with 10 respondents from the Psychopharmacology Task Force Educational Survey who indicated on the survey that they used computer-assisted technology to teach psychopharmacology.

Findings

Interactive Videos: There were no interactive video programs on psychopharmacology available commercially.

Computer-Assisted Instruction: There is one comprehensive program, "Med Clinic," available from Computerized Educational Systems (1-800-275-1474). It simulates decisions about assessment data and interventions in a "Community Mental Health Center Medication Clinic." It is directed at the generalist level of nursing practice.

There are two programs specific to psychiatric disorders by Medi-Sim (1-800-527-5597). One covers inpatient psychotropic treatment of a young schizophrenic man and is somewhat outdated. The other one covers inpatient treatment of a depressed woman with tricyclic antidepressants.

Medi-Sim also has a computer series available in four separate programs which cover psychopharmacology broadly: "Introduction to Drug Therapy," "Systems of Measurement," and "Medication Administration, Parts 1 and 2." These programs review drug terminology, roles of health team members, medication orders, nursing responsibilities, and documentation, and they are directed at the basic nursing student.*

---

*The American Nurses Association and American Nurses Foundation neither endorse nor recommend use of these products.

Videotapes: There were no nursing-generated videotapes for psychopharmacology located. A review of available videos for psychiatry revealed that most of them are outdated. There also were no nursing-generated brain biology videos located.

Summary

Despite the advanced media technology available today, there are few offerings in the computer/video industry in psychopharmacology and related neurosciences for psychiatric nurses.

Psychiatric Nursing Conferences

Mary Ann Nihart, M.A., R.N.

A convenience sample of 35 national psychiatric mental health nursing conferences held from 1987 through 1992 was obtained from inquiries made of psychiatric nurse leaders and requests made to national sponsors.

This review includes 35 conferences: 11 conferences sponsored by national psychiatric nursing organizations—Association of Child and Adolescent Psychiatric Nurses (ACAPN), American Psychiatric Nurses Association (APNA), and Society for Education and Research in Psychiatric-Mental Health Nursing (SERPN); 19 organized by nationally oriented nursing education sponsors such as Contemporary Forums, Nursing Transitions, and Resource Applications; and five held independently but advertised to a national audience.

Conference locations were distributed throughout the nation (Table 19). Small regional or local conferences targeting smaller geographical areas were not included in this review.

A qualitative review of conference programs was completed, based on presentation title and knowledge of the presenter's focus. These presentations were then placed in the following categories:

1. General psychopharmacology (medication administration, side effects, clinical management);
2. Neurobiology (neuro-anatomy, neurophysiology, related neurosciences);
3. Other related topics (prescriptive authority, medication informed consent).

Some presentations were difficult to categorize because published titles may not have reflected psychopharmacological or biological content and the presenters could not be contacted. As a result, some relevant presentations may have been overlooked.

Table 20 provides percentages of total hours of presentation for each topic included in the conferences reviewed. Although this analysis has significant limitations—such as convenience sampling, difficulty in categorizing presentations, and unavailability of content for all years analyzed—some trends are suggested from the available information.

TABLE 19

Conference Report by Location

NORTHEAST/EAST - 10	SOUTHEAST - 7	MIDWEST - 5	CENTRAL/SOUTH - 4	WEST - 9
Baltimore	Atlanta	Chicago	Dallas	Denver
Washington, DC	Orlando	Indianapolis	New Orleans	San Francisco
White Plains, NY	Hilton Head, SC	Kansas City		Palm Springs
Atlantic City	Williamsburg, VA			Las Vegas
Philadelphia	Lexington, KY			Anaheim
Boston				San Diego
Stanford, CT				Honolulu

TABLE 20

Percent of Presentations at Conferences by Topic

CONFERENCES	1992 %P	1992 %B	1991 %P	1991 %B	1990 %P	1990 %B	1989 %P	1989 %B
ACAPN	2.32/0	0	6.25/0	0	0	4.78	2.27/0	0
APNA	6.52/0	0	N/A	N/A	6.52/0	3.26	6.35/0	1.59
SERPN	0/5.13	14.10	6.12/0	23.33	0	2.32	N/A	N/A
CONT FORUMS EAST WEST	21.16/ 3.17 23.28/0	6.35 7.40	18.63/0 14.91/0	7.45 5.59	13.12/0 5.63/0	1.88 7.50	5.63/0 3.75/0	0 3.75
NSG TRAN	0	3.42	11.73/0	10.06	2.15/0	3.00	3.25/0	3.90
RES APPL EAST WEST SOUTH	9.05/0 1.65/0 9.05/0	5.24 5.83 5.24	9.35/0 4.11/0 N/A	10.75 0 N/A	5.91/0 N/A 8.56/0	9.14 N/A 5.35	N/A N/A N/A	N/A N/A N/A

Note: Total conference hours included all concurrent sessions. Some topics were repeated.
%P = % Psychopharmacology/% Psychopharmacology-Related Topics; %B = Biology-Related Topics.
N/A = Not available or was not conducted.

Findings

There has been an increase in conference time spent on biological issues and psychopharmacology. Below are the mean percentages for each year.

	1989	1990	1991	1992
Biological issues:	1.85%	4.65%	8.17%	5.29%
Psychopharmacology:	4.25%	5.24%	8.89%	11.44%

Overall, this represents a threefold to fivefold increase in emphasis on these topics.

Information was collected from conversations with conference coordinators. This review suggests that interest in and demand for psychopharmacology and related neurosciences have also increased, as evidenced by the increased popularity of pre-conferences and specialty topics in these fields.

Review of conferences prior to 1989 suggests the percentages for that year are representative of most conferences during the late 1980s. It is also important to note that there is a significantly greater increase in independent conferences than in those sponsored by psychiatric nursing organizations. These independent sponsors market primarily to the staff nurse and clinical nurse specialist levels of practice.

A review of presentation content reveals that psychopharmacology topics have become more specific to diagnostic groups and subclasses of medications. For example, the most common presentation in the late 1980s was a general psychopharmacology update while in 1992 the following topics were more common:

Biological Topics

- Biological psychiatry and the future of psychiatric nursing;
- The neurophysiology of anger;
- Biological rhythm disturbances in depression and rhythm-specific nursing;
- Biological measures in the treatment of depression; and,
- Information processing deficits in the treatment of schizophrenia.

Psychopharmacology Topics

- Atypical antipsychotics: Nursing interventions and the application of the biology of schizophrenia;
- Integrating psychodynamics and psychopharmacology in the treatment of borderline personalities;

- Patterns of PRN medication use in response to aggressive behavior; and,
- Serotonin-selective antidepressants and suicidality.

However, with this shift there is also evidence of increased utilization of non-nursing presenters, such as physicians and pharmacists.

In 1991 and 1992, several individual conferences focused entirely on biological information. Some provided basic neuroscience information, while others offered research presentations and applications to psychiatric nursing (Table 20). The presentation of topics in biological issues related to psychiatry at more broadly focused conferences also suggests a need for basic information as well as more sophisticated application of basic neurosciences for psychiatric nursing.

Summary

The greater emphasis on biological and psychopharmacological topics in the national psychiatric nursing conferences surveyed provides strong evidence of the increasing interest in and need for information in these areas. Despite these trends, however, psychiatric nursing conferences are not the only source of information on these topics. Many nurses also attend interdisciplinary educational offerings and numerous local workshops, making the actual need for this information more difficult to assess.

National Psychopharmacology Conference: The Practice Perspective

A National Conference for Competencies in Psychopharmacology for Psychiatric Mental Health Nurses was held at ANA Headquarters in Washington, D.C. in spring 1993. The purpose of this two-day working conference was to assess the practice settings for psychiatric mental health nurses in relation to working with patients receiving psychopharmacologic treatment for their mental illness. Conference participants were nominated by their state nurses associations (SNAs) at the request of ANA.

One hundred and seventy applications were received, and final selections were made to ensure representation by region of the country, race, gender, educational preparation, area of practice, and expertise in psychopharmacology. The list of conference attendees is presented in Appendix 1.

The keynote address, *Efficacy of Major Psychotropic Medications: Critical Role for Nursing*, was delivered by Jeanne Miller Fox, Ph.D., R.N., F.A.A.N., a national leader in psychiatric mental health nursing. A summary of her report is presented in Appendix 3.

The Psychopharmacology Task Force presented the findings of the nursing environment review on educational content, publications and resources, computer resources and videos, and conferences.

Several consumer participants presented a panel discussion, *Persons Experiencing the Effects of Mental Disorders*, which included their perspective on what consumers of mental health services would like psychiatric nurses to know about medication from the patient and family perspective. A summary of their presentation is included in Appendix 4.

These presentations set an enlightened and inspired tone for the work of the conference. Participants selected one of five conference work groups corresponding to the content areas initially identified by the task force as guides for organizing psychopharmacologic content for psychiatric nurses: *neurosciences, clinical psychopharmacology, clinical assessment, clinical management, and legal/ethical issues*. Each of these work groups was facilitated by members of the task force.

The consensus of each work group was presented to the conference as a whole in several summary sessions during the conference. The resultant feedback and exchange of ideas helped cultivate and refine the work of each group. Final summaries and recommendations from each group for nursing practice in psychopharmacology and related neurosciences were synthesized by task force members and are presented herein.

Neurosciences: Developing a Basic Science Foundation for Psychiatric Nurses

Norman L. Keltner, Ed.D., R.N.
Gloria B. Callwood, Ph.D., R.N.

Historically, in non-psychiatric nursing specialty areas, patient care has been well grounded in basic science. Moreover, this knowledge has been viewed as a prerequisite to practice and fundamental to effective treatment. This same emphasis has not traditionally held true for the psychiatric nursing specialty. In psychiatric nursing, historical, philosophical, and political issues converged to create a climate in which psychiatric nurses knew little about neurobiological factors, were not encouraged to obtain this knowledge, and oftentimes viewed neurobiological explanations and treatments as falling outside the domain of nursing practice.

By contrast, other disciplines, especially medicine and psychology, have begun to focus on the new technologies and theories provided recently by the rapidly expanding neurosciences. Instead, psychiatric nursing, until recently, has had a nearly exclusive focus on psychodynamic and behavioral theories as unidimensional explanations of mental illness.

The practical results of such a knowledge deficit for psychiatric nurses in the current scientific milieu are a restricted participation in clinical care, less than optimum treatment of patients with mental illness, and limited leadership opportunities in the field of mental health. During this "Decade of the Brain," many psychiatric nurses are recognizing the importance of neuroscientific findings and are requesting this information.

For example, brain imaging technology is penetrating barriers never before breached and providing unprecedented information about how the human brain functions. If one is not well grounded in basic brain science, such findings cannot be understood or integrated into the design, implementation, or measurement of standard or innovative psychiatric interventions.

A working knowledge of basic brain biology is fundamental to understanding theoretical frameworks for mental disorders, brain imaging technology, and psychopharmacology. Nursing models that benefit patients with psychiatric disorders must account for the biologic basis of mental illness. And to comprehend much of the current psychiatric research literature, one must have a firm grasp of brain biology to interpret findings regarding human behavior and psychiatric interventions.

In addition, the longer nursing delays in soundly encompassing the cutting-edge information provided by the neurosciences, the more difficult it will be to master information that increases almost daily, and is fast becoming the basis for the entire field of mental health.

TABLE 21

Neuroscience Content for Psychiatric Nurses

I. Neuro-anatomy

Cerebrum
Thalamus
Limbic System
Basal Ganglia
Cranial Nerves
Hemispheres and Lobes of the Brain

Cerebellum
Hypothalamus Reticular System
Corpus Callosum
Brain Stem

Peripheral Nervous System (PNS)
Extrapyramidal System (EPS)
Neuronal Structure and Function

II. Genetic/Familial Correlates

Genetic structures
    RNA
    DNA
    Chromosomes
Principles of Genetic Investigation
    Familial Aggregation Studies
    Twin and Adoption Studies
    Segregation Analysis
    Genetic Linkage

III. Systems of Neuroregulation

Neurotransmitters
    1. Amino Acids   3. Acetylcholine
    2. Monoamines   4. Neuropeptides
Enzymes
Cellular neurochemistry/electrophysiology in neurotransmission

IV. Psychoendocrinology

Hypothalamic - Pituitary - Thyroid Axis (HPT)
Hypothalamic - Pituitary - Adrenal Axis (HPA)
Hypothalamic - Pituitary - Gonadal Axis (HPG)

V. Psychoimmunology

Basic components of the Immune System
    Lymph nodes   Phagocytes
    Bone marrow   Leukocytes
Stress response mechanisms
    Differential effects of Long-Term Stress vs. Short-Term Stress
    Catacholamines
    Cortisol

VI. Normal Biological Rhythms

Sleep-Wake
Temperature
Hormonal

VII. Psychobiological Dysfunctions

Kindling
Sleep Disturbances
Biological Rhythm Changes

VIII. Biological Theories of Major Psychiatric Disorders

Schizophrenia
Anxiety Disorders
Substance Abuse
Seizure Disorders
Tourette's Syndrome

Mood Disorders
Personality Disorders
Delirium/Dementias
Trauma/Infection
Obsessive-Compulsive Disorder

IX. Brain Imaging in Diagnosis of Mental Illness

Computerized Tomography (CT)
Magnetic Resonance Imaging (MRI)
Positron Emission Tomography (PET)
Single Photon Emission Computerized Tomography (SPECT)

X. Physiological Indices of Mental Illness

Laboratory Studies

Furthermore, incomplete understanding of basic neuroscience will make it difficult for psychiatric nurses to thoroughly represent such approaches as wellness or holism, concepts that may be important for a truly integrated approach to health care. Theoretical models such as wellness or holism are poorly researched to date, difficult to measure, and as yet ungrounded in scientific theory. Utilizing such models without the ability to integrate and articulate possible neuroscientific explanations or design neuroscientific studies is to psychiatric nursings' professional disadvantage.

Balance

Psychiatric mental health nursing is faced with the difficult task of designing methods to incorporate neuroscientific information throughout the specialty. Each individual psychiatric mental health nurse, educational program, and practice setting must strike a balance between important and traditional practice parameters and new scientific information.

To set a goal of mid-level knowledge may be more readily achievable but may not be sufficiently far-reaching. On the other hand, to set too high a standard too soon risks a greater likelihood for failure.

Further content mastery for all psychiatric nurses is realistically a re-education process. Such a process will be expensive and time-consuming. The very practical issues such as who will teach, who will supervise, are significant problems to address, but every step toward this end is a valuable one.

Table 21 provides a list of content areas developed by the neuroscience conference work group during the National Psychopharmacology Conference. The work group felt that this information was fundamental to the care of patients with mental illness, and, thus, to the specialty of psychiatric nursing.

Clinical Psychopharmacology: Considerations for Nursing Practice

Mary Ann Nihart, M.A., R.N.
Michele T. Laraia, R.N., M.S.N.

Psychiatric mental health nurses administer and monitor psychopharmacologic agents, and educate individuals with psychiatric disorders and their families about them. The task of the psychopharmacology conference work group was to identify the information needed to perform these functions effectively. Solid expertise in the area of clinical psychopharmacology was one essential that immediately became evident as the work group began discussions of what information should be included.

During the initial working session, the group members generated long lists of specific information related to all aspects of clinical psychopharmacology. The global topics discussed included:

- Pharmacokinetics and pharmacodynamics
- Target symptoms
- Stages and progression of illness
- Factors affecting medication choice
- Development of treatment plans
- Medication effect variables
- Drug interactions and side effects
- Monitoring
- Psycho-education
- Quality of life
- Discontinuation
- Relapse prevention
- Continuing education

Further discussion in this work group led to a renewed appreciation for the breadth of knowledge required by all nurses who are involved in any aspect of treatment utilizing psychopharmacologic agents. It became evident that several key questions needed to be addressed:

- What medications should be considered psychopharmacologic agents?
- What disorders are being treated with these medications?
- At what levels of practice do psychiatric nurses perform the various functions of clinical psychopharmacology?
- What specific information needs to be covered?
- How should information about clinical psychopharmacology be organized?

■ How can psychiatric nurses be assisted in acquiring and maintaining knowledge and skill in psychopharmacology?

Medications to Be Included

All medications used for psychotherapeutic indications were considered. Obviously, medications such as antipsychotics, antidepressants, antimanics, anxiolytics, and sedative/hypnotics should be included. However, recognizing that some medications used for psychiatric purposes—such as carbamazepine, valproate, and propranolol—have not traditionally been classified as psychiatric drugs, all medications used for psychotherapeutic indications were considered. The work group concluded that psychiatric nurses at all levels of practice must be well informed about the use of these medications for illnesses defined in the latest *Diagnostic and Statistical Manual (DSM)* (APA 1994).

Well-informed psychiatric nurses, regardless of practice level, distinguish between the physiological actions, therapeutic effects, side effects, and approved indications of the various psychopharmacologic agents as well as uses outside of approved indications. Psychiatric nurses at all levels of practice must also have the knowledge about medications used for relief of side effects caused by psychopharmacologic agents, and psychiatric symptoms of medical disorders.

Treatment Indications and Level of Practice

The work group agreed that psychotherapeutic indications included treatment of a variety of psychiatric disorders reflected in the latest *DSM*. Various taxonomies of nursing diagnoses, such as the North American Nursing Diagnostic Association (NANDA), add important patient-specific characteristics that guide the nurse in the overall therapeutic approach to patients, including, in some instances, psychopharmacologic interventions.

Because the psychiatric nurse is educated at both the undergraduate and graduate levels, there is a continuum of knowledge concerning the use of psychopharmacologic agents, as well as psychiatric nursing interventions. For any given psychiatric nurse, depending on level of education and clinical experience, knowledge will range on this continuum from the observation of global behavioral responses to psychopharmacologic agents to a level of specificity that is cellular.

Whether administering or monitoring medications, or educating patients and their families about medications, or fulfilling the role of advanced practice clinicians, psychiatric nurses carry out nursing functions commensurate with their level of practice. This level of practice is based on educational preparation, experience, clinical setting, credentialing, and licensing.

Continued discussions by the psychopharmacology work group led to the identification of special populations requiring additional knowledge on the part of the nurse for safe and appropriate use of psychopharmacologic agents. These populations are "special" because they have particular needs based on age, gender, or other biological, social, cultural, or economic parameters.

They may have belief systems that influence the effectiveness of treatment. They may belong to segments of the population that have been under-represented in psychopharmacologic clinical studies, thus, less may be known about the effects of drug treatment in these groups.

Racial and ethnic/cultural diversity as well as gender and socioeconomic factors can influence an individual's response to psychopharmacologic medications. The psychiatric nurse must be aware of the potential influence of each of these factors and perform assessments, develop treatment plans, and anticipate outcomes based on this knowledge.

These special populations include but are not limited to: children, the elderly, pregnant women, individuals with developmental disorders, and individuals with concurrent health considerations.

Information and Organization

With each medication chosen for use, the psychopharmacology work group agreed that the nurse must have the knowledge and experience to develop a psychopharmacologic treatment plan commensurate with level of practice. This treatment plan should be based on knowledge of psychopharmacologic agents, patient assessment, and phase of treatment, and can be used to organize patient-specific information regarding psycho-pharmacologic intervention.

PSYCHOPHARMACOLOGIC ASSESSMENT

The nurse should know the following information about each drug being used:

- Medication actions;
- Target effects;
- Unwanted effects, such as side effects, toxicity, and adverse effects;
- Medication management, such as dosage, scheduling, lab monitoring, symptom assessment;
- Precautions/contraindications; and,
- Interactive effects, such as with other medications, food, health status, behavior, and the environment.

PATIENT ASSESSMENT

The nurse should know the following patient-specific information:

- Baseline target symptom assessment, including the use of standardized rating scales;
- Assessment of concurrent substance use, including alcohol, illicit drugs, nicotine, over-the-counter medications, and caffeine;
- Assessment of appropriate patient variables, such as demographic, physical, socioeconomic, past experiences, and patient and family preferences and beliefs; and,
- Use of physical, lab, mental status, and diagnostic assessments.

PHASE OF TREATMENT

Although assessment is ongoing and, thus, may overlap with subsequent treatment phases, organizing treatment in terms of phases provides a framework for the psychiatric nurse. This framework facilitates the use of complex and changing information encountered in the treatment of individuals with psychiatric disorders. Modifications to the treatment plan may be necessary at any point in the course of treatment. However, these phases offer points at which adjustments in psychopharmacologic management may most often occur.

The following is a list of clinical considerations in each of four treatment phases:

Initiation

- Pharmacokinetics/Pharmacodynamics
- Client education about medication and alternative treatments
- Informed consent
- Identification of target symptoms and rating scales
- Early medication effects
- Alternative treatments
- Development of treatment plans
- Implications of information obtained in assessment

Stabilization

- Continued assessment of target symptoms
- Expected timing of medication effects
- Recognition and treatment of adverse effects
- Therapeutic drug monitoring
- When and how to change medication strategies
- Ongoing patient education
- Transition between treatment settings

Maintenance

- Education regarding relapse and recognition of stressors
- Monitoring efficacy, side effects, and laboratory values
- Consider long-term side effect potential
- Address compliance issues
- When and how to discontinue medication treatment
- Patient education for relapse prevention

Medication-Free

- Duration of treatment for a given disorder
- Tapering methods/schedules
- Symptom recognition
- Relapse prevention

Acquisition of Knowledge and Continuing Education

Recognizing the breadth of knowledge required in psychopharmacology, the work group turned to a lengthy discussion of how new graduates and psychiatric mental health nurses currently in practice, education, and research can acquire this complex information and remain up-to-date.

The work group endorsed the need for psychopharmacology to be included in all levels of nursing education, practice, and research. This knowledge should build upon information in nursing education and must be integrated at the clinical level. Nurse researchers should consider integrating neuroscientific information into nursing theory development, research protocols, and publications.

The work group discussed the need for more adjunctive educational materials, improved textbooks, more journal and newsletter coverage, and availability of psychopharmacological databases. The work group concluded that it is each psychiatric nurse's responsibility to develop a plan for continued education in psychopharmacology and related neurosciences.

Clinical Assessment in Contemporary Nursing Practice

Lawrence Scahill, R.N., M.S.N., M.P.H.
Sandra Talley, M.N., R.N., A.N.P.

Assessment includes systematic collection of data, identification of primary problems, and evaluation of therapeutic intervention with modification of treatment goals as necessary. Clinical specialty provides additional direction concerning the nature of data to be collected and ways of conceptualizing presenting problems.

The recent advances in psychiatry with respect to nosology and neurobiology of mental illness have tremendous implications for psychiatric nursing practice at all levels, both in terms of assessment and treatment. These implications are especially pertinent to nursing practice in psychopharmacology.

Among the first issues to be settled in defining assessment in contemporary psychiatric nursing was the differentiation of basic versus advanced level of practice. In developing these guidelines for clinical assessment, the assessment conference work group of clinicians and educators concluded that the differentiation between levels of nursing practice is primarily a matter of depth.

Thus, several domains of assessment were deemed appropriate for both generalists in psychiatric mental health nursing and advanced practice psychiatric clinical nurse specialists. These domains include: physical, psychiatric, psychopharmacological, and environmental areas.

This summary of the conference work group on assessment briefly describes these four areas of assessment and provides some guidance concerning the clinical implications for basic and advanced levels of nursing practice.

Physical Assessment

Physical assessment is relevant to psychiatric nursing for several reasons. First, some physical disorders can be accompanied by psychiatric symptoms and some psychiatric disorders can result in physiologic complications. In addition, a substantial percentage of those with severe mental illness do not have access to primary health care services. The health status of patients prior to starting pharmacotherapy and over the course of treatment may influence the selection and continuation of psychopharmacologic agents.

Psychiatric nursing practice at the basic level includes:

- General techniques of physical assessment such as inspection, observation, measurement of vital signs;
- Review of laboratory data; and,
- Survey of health history.

Nurses with advanced training may be prepared to conduct a thorough physical examination, review of systems, and health history.

Finally, specific diagnostic procedures may be indicated for certain psychopharmacologic agents or for particular patient populations.

Psychiatric Assessment

Data for psychiatric assessment accrue from several sources:

- Patient interview
- Clinical observation
- Reports of family members
- Reports of significant others (e.g., teachers, clergy, and health care providers)

The clinical interview, like the physical examination, becomes progressively more sophisticated with the nurse's experience and guided learning. Components of the psychiatric assessment include:

- the patient's chief complaint
- history of present problem
- past treatment history
- mental status examination
- personality structure and coping style
- review of past treatment records.

Clearly, the ability to conduct a systematic and comprehensive psychiatric assessment depends on education and clinical experience. However, all nurses practicing in psychiatric settings should be capable of making fundamental judgments about the patient's level of consciousness, appearance, speech, affect, and social relatedness. Nurses with advanced training in psychiatric nursing will be able to conduct a full psychiatric assessment leading to diagnosis and a comprehensive treatment plan.

Standardized clinical rating scales are useful to confirm or question diagnoses objectively and to measure symptom severity. Baseline ratings can also be useful as comparisons against how to evaluate change in symptom severity following the initiation of therapeutic interventions. Training and experience are required to achieve valid and reliable ratings. However, acquaintance with the types and applications of commonly used standardized clinical rating scales will become increasingly important for all nurses working in psychiatric settings.

Pharmacological Assessment

Comprehensive physical and psychiatric assessments ideally converge and form the basis of intervention, including psychopharmacological intervention. Areas to be considered in psychopharmacological assessment include:

- Target symptoms and selection of treatment methods
- Side-effect profile of selected pharmacologic agents
- Response to prior medication
- Concomitant drug use
- Drug allergies
- Patient preference for treatment
- Therapeutic response of first-degree (biological) family members to medication for related problems.

Baseline data about allergies, concomitant drug use, and previous response to drug therapy are fundamental guides to treatment planning. For example, drug choices within a specific drug category (antipsychotics or antidepressants) can be resolved by considering previous drug response, adverse effects, and allergies. Similarly, a thorough understanding of concurrent medical treatment is essential because some medical treatments may interact with psychopharmacological interventions.

A recognized useful predictor of drug response is also the therapeutic response of first-degree (biological) family members. As more is learned about the genetics of psychiatric illness in terms of receptor subtypes, regulation of functionally related brain pathways, and synthesis of neurotransmitters, family psychiatric history, including drug response, will be more helpful.

Environmental Assessment

An extension of the chief complaint is the patient's stated or unstated goal of treatment. Exploration of the chief complaint often leads to the identification of the patient's hope for treatment with certain goals in mind, goals which may or may not be consistent with that of the family or significant others in the patient's environment. Moreover, the patient's and family's goals for treatment, whether consistent or not, may go beyond what is realistic.

Environmental assessment considers the patient's:

- household composition and support systems
- education, occupation, and financial circumstances
- ethnicity and cultural heritage
- lifestyle

Environmental factors can influence treatment planning in several ways. For example, financial strain might have an impact on treatment compliance if the medication of choice is expensive. Cultural heritage may affect the patient and family attitude toward mental illness and the use of medication. Identification and negotiation of these issues may be critical to the success or failure of a psychopharmacological intervention.

Another important component of environmental assessment is the context of care, including other health care providers and treatment settings. Obviously, nurses in psychiatric settings must cultivate a collaborative relationship with other professionals. In addition, plans for follow-up care should consider not only what is available but also what is acceptable to the patient and the family. Matching the patient's preferences with available resources is the goal of environmental assessment.

Conclusions

Clinical assessment in contemporary psychiatric nursing is influenced by training, experience, and setting. Nonetheless, several principles endure regardless of the level of training. First, clinical assessment is collaborative and includes the findings and impressions from interdisciplinary team members as well as health care colleagues and family members and available community support systems.

Secondly, sound clinical judgment requires the integration of findings from physical, psychiatric, pharmacological, and environmental domains. Finally, expertise in clinical assessment relies on formal education, clinical experience, and supervised training, and entails moving beyond collecting and recording data to processing the meaning of the data gathered.

Guiding Principles in the Clinical Management of Psychopharmacology

Linda S. Beeber, Ph.D., R.N.
Jeanne Anne Clement, Ed.D., R.N.
Susan Simmons-Alling, M.S.N., R.N.

In the practice of psychiatric mental health nursing, the goal of clinical management of psychopharmacologic interventions is to promote physiological stability that will permit the attainment of psychological, social, and spiritual growth—thus enhancing the quality of the patient's life and health. The psychiatric nurse achieves this through the creation of a patient-focused treatment system that utilizes the benefits of psychopharmacologic agents to the patient's best advantage.

The psychiatric nurse forms a partnership with the patient and significant others to create a mental health treatment system that empowers the individual to regulate psychopharmacologic interventions in a manner that is in harmony with his or her life. For the psychiatric nurse, clinical management of psychopharmacologic agents requires the synthesis of knowledge, experience, and clinical skill, as well as the authority and responsibility to manage and facilitate psychopharmacologic treatment.

This section provides a conceptual approach to the clinical management of patients receiving psychopharmacologic agents. Key elements in the clinical management of patients receiving psychopharmacologic interventions are:

- Ecological advocacy
- Collaboration
- Efficacy and progress of treatment
- Education
- Legal and ethical standards.

Ecological Advocacy

Ecological advocacy includes the process as well as the philosophical perspective taken by the psychiatric nurse to assure that psychopharmacologic interventions fit with the overall style and quality of the patient's life. This process is interactive and requires working with patients and their significant others to clarify individual interpretations of what constitutes quality of life.

Interaction between nurse and patient includes both the acquisition and the provision of information from a variety of sources. Information from the psychiatric nurse includes that gained during clinical assessment, and from other sources, that will, in turn, provide guidelines for use of that information. The information equips the patient with the resources needed to preserve the essential tenets of quality of life and the ability to integrate psychopharmacologic treatment and the important activities of life.

For example, in the case where psychopharmacologic agents are effective for the target symptoms suffered by the patient, but where side effects hinder meaningful work or pleasure, the psychiatric nurse will help the patient evaluate and manipulate treatment effects through education, changing medication strategies, or even supporting the discontinuation of psychopharmacologic treatment. Acquisition of information by the nurse comes from careful and respectful listening to the patient, significant others, other providers, as well as that gained by formal education and clinical experience.

Ecological advocacy requires the management of psychopharmacologic agents in a manner that integrates them with other interventions to the patient's best advantage. One example of this is in situations where gravely altered levels of function or behavior have threatened the stability of the patient's support system. Often, situations such as this require a comprehensive look at all appropriate interventions, including psychopharmacology. Interventions which accomplish alteration of the environment, both emotional and physical, may be necessary to achieve integration between the patient and support systems.

Ecological advocacy also requires that the psychiatric nurse exercise power and skill in the creation of a patient-focused health care delivery system. A patient-focused system is responsive to the immediate and long-term needs of the individual and significant others in dimensions of time, location, and cost. A patient-focused system meets the needs of a culturally competent plural patient population. To engage in the process of ecological advocacy, the psychiatric nurse collaborates, monitors treatment effectiveness and progress, and maintains legal and ethical standards.

Collaboration

Collaboration is the process of achieving goals through joint effort. Inherent in this process is equality among the collaborators, each one bringing unique and essen-

tial skills to the process. For the patient, entry into the mental health care system usually requires a special effort to achieve collaborative status, and advocacy for the patient is frequently necessary to maintain individual dignity and self-esteem. Some patients may find it difficult to negotiate authentic collaboration with the health care system as equal partners and knowledgeable consumers of services.

Nurses can serve as advocates for patients by facilitating a collaborative environment. Open and free exchange of information, mutual recognition of expertise, and shared power and authority characterize successful collaboration.

The process of collaboration is integral to the process of ecological advocacy. In collaboration, differences of perception are reconciled among patient, family, and provider systems. Differences in perceptions belie different, and at times, contradictory needs and values. These differences need to be identified and made explicit, as failure to resolve conflicts in individual and system needs or values is at the heart of most unilateral treatment decisions or treatment interruptions.

Initiation of and continued use of psychopharmacologic agents involve making choices that change as the individual grows and develops, and as life events occur. As the patient makes choices collaboratively with the nurse and the other members of the health care team, the nurse must make a commitment to "live through the choice with the patient." This commitment may mean maintaining a supportive and trusting relationship with the patient who chooses a direction that is different from that advocated by the nurse and/or the treatment team. At times, this means advocating for these choices with other providers and significant others.

Efficacy and Progress of Treatment

An effective psychopharmacologic treatment program begins with collaboration with the patient and significant others to develop an agreed upon plan of care with the goal of agreed upon outcomes. This requires the development of diagnostic reliability in both the medical and nursing spheres.

Once a recommendation for treatment has been made, the choice of medication must be integrated with the patient's perspective on significant life issues, and initiation of psychopharmacologic agents is done by balancing side effects and efficacy as appropriate.

Efficacy and progress of treatment require the management of dosages collaboratively with the patient to establish "adjustment ranges" within which the patient can alter the dosage pattern. Other predetermined agreements with the patient—and significant others where appropriate—and part of the agreed upon plan, include processes for handling missed doses and physiological conditions that require a change in dosage.

Progress must be measured over a sufficient period of time and should include consistent monitoring of the medication against the chosen target symptoms. Consideration should be given to the overall functioning of the patient, patient satisfaction, and self-care practices.

Continual monitoring must be done for adverse effects that may occur over the course of psychopharmacologic treatment. Monitoring processes should also include screening for factors that interfere with the actions of the medication and/or the monitoring process itself.

The psychiatric nurse must know the general principles of interactions as well as specific medication interactions with foods, other drugs, and environmental influences and the influence of age. For psychopharmacology to be as effective as possible, side effects as well as the patient's idiosyncratic responses to medications must be identified and treated. Monitoring is an unending process, particularly in disorders characterized by remissions and exacerbations.

Monitoring the course of illness and the effects of psychopharmacologic agents requires the use of standardized measures, such as behavioral rating scales, that are reliable and valid, and the development of systematic methods where objective measures are not appropriate or available. In particular, there is a need to develop practical, systematic methods of tracking side effects and recognizing adverse effects.

Maintaining efficacy requires the psychiatric nurse to develop a response plan, in conjunction with the patient and significant others, that is quick and sensitive to changes in the patient's symptom status. This strategy includes defining conditions requiring changes in dosages or medications, and the identification of additional and alternative avenues of intervention. Finally, efficacy requires working with the patient and significant others to create advance directives which are the agreed upon actions to be taken when the patient's decision making ability is compromised by symptoms.

Education

At the heart of ecological advocacy is patient education. Education should be offered in a manner in which the patient is fully informed regarding care, and assumes ownership, gives consent, and uses the knowledge to direct the process of pharmacotherapy. Patients and significant others need to know about the disorder, its symptoms, and psychopharmacologic treatments, as well as concurrent and alternative treatment modalities. Issues of long-term importance such as new knowledge about biological correlates of mental symptoms, genetics, short- and long-term dangers of medication therapy, and information necessary to make informed life decisions must be addressed.

Education must include preparation of the patient in self-medication. This requires going beyond the initiation phase to the provision of supports that assist the patient in becoming maximally involved in self-medication. This includes outreach systems that provide in-home assistance when necessary and community-based services. Education also includes strategies that help the patient minimize the obvious signs of taking medication that could contribute to the stigma often accompanying mental illness.

To be proficient at teaching patients and their significant others, psychiatric nurses must be knowledgeable about psychopharmacology and principles of education. The nurse must be able to assess learning styles in patients and their families, and be able to vary techniques in response to these assessed qualities. Developmental levels, reading ability, and multi-linguistic/multicultural factors must be integrated into the preparation of materials and media. Education must include documentation of learning as well as of teaching, evidence of what the patient knows, and documentation of how and when the patient's knowledge is changed by symptoms of the disorder.

Legal and Ethical Standards

Ecological advocacy in the clinical management of psychopharmacological interventions includes the development of and adherence to clear and reasonable standards of mental health practice. Collaborative decision making, informed consent, and advance directives are essential components of the highest standards of legal and ethical mental health care.

Legal and Ethical Issues Related to Psychopharmacology

Susan Caverly, M.A., R.N.

This work group was charged with identifying the salient legal and ethical issues in psychiatric nursing with respect to psychopharmacology. Because legal issues and ethical issues are not one and the same, legal and ethical dimensions will be reviewed separately.

Legal Requirements

Legal requirements related to psychopharmacologic practice for nurses rest in the realm of knowledge acquisition and maintenance. Specifically, this refers to knowledge of the minimal requirement for licensure and regulation in the state in which the nurse practices. These requirements can be different from those of the institution in which the nurse works and the nurse is expected to understand that the regulatory requirements supersede those of the institution. The nurse is required to maintain current knowledge of the state law related to nursing practice, and is responsible for acting within the parameters of that law.

The following parameters represent what the psychiatric nurse is legally obligated to ensure:

- that any prescriptive orders followed are within the legal parameters of the state law and the scope of practice of the authority from which the orders derive. This legal authority prescribing party may be a nurse or a professional from another discipline.
- that informed consent for pharmacologic treatment has been obtained prior to prescribing or administering the medication.
- that documentation of patient assessment and treatment is included in the clinical record. This information should document medication side effects, compliance, patient education, effectiveness, identification of target symptoms, referral of treatment responsibility or consultation, and, when applicable, differential diagnoses.
- that patient consent is obtained prior to release of confidential information related to psychopharmacologic treatment. In the event of emergency, this obligation may be superseded (depending on state law) by the need to provide an emergency practitioner with the information necessary to treat the patient.

- that the administration of, or when appropriate to level of practice, the prescription of the correct medication in the appropriate dose is given to the right patient.
- that the nurse understands, monitors, and records effects of the medication administered or prescribed.
- that whenever tasks are delegated to a non-nurse care giver, the individual possesses the knowledge, skill, and ability to perform the appropriate tasks related to the psychopharmacologic intervention and to monitor the outcome of the intervention.

Ethical Obligations

Although salient ethical issues were easily identified by the work group, establishing consensus regarding the hierarchy of issues and application of ethical principles in individual cases was more difficult. This difficulty led to much discussion regarding level of practice and preparation for practice. Among the dimensions of ethical obligations—for the psychiatric mental health nurse—related to psychopharmacology, are the concepts of benefit, autonomy, best interest and contextual factors, research, and nursing actions regarding negligence or malpractice (Jonsen et al. 1992). Each of these issues will be described briefly.

Benefit refers to the perceived or expected benefit of treatment and the medical indication of a specific treatment.

Knowledge is considered an ethical obligation. Because psychiatric nurses are directly involved in psychopharmacologic treatment of patients with mental illness, nurses are obligated to obtain and maintain current knowledge of basic psychopharmacology. Psychiatric nurses also have an obligation to ascertain the symptoms of mental illness that are likely to respond to psychopharmacologic interventions, as well as contraindications and potential side effects of those interventions.

There is an ethical obligation to determine what information is relevant and requires that it be written in the medical record to facilitate clinical review for the appropriateness and efficacy of psychopharmacologic intervention.

Autonomy refers to patient preference regarding choice of care or treatment and the ability to exercise this choice without undue pressure.

An ethical obligation exists that requires psychiatric nurses to continue working with a patient or to provide reasonable referral when appropriate. When the patient exercises the right to refuse psychopharmacologic treatment, psychiatric nurses are obligated to explain, or provide or refer for alternative treatments.

Relevant aspects in this area include:

- To offer only those psychopharmacologic agents which are clinically indicated;
- To continue to offer or recommend psychopharmacologic treatment and document the patient's refusal; and,
- To provide ongoing assessment of the patient's ability to function and to discuss the risks and benefits of initiating psychopharmacological treatment for the time the patient is under the care of the nurse.

Best interests refers to the ethical obligation to act in the best interests of the patient. Some examples:

- Provision of information related to consent for psychopharmacological treatment that matches the patient's ability to understand;
- Recognition that there are times in the course of mental illness when the patient's own capacity to make decisions is impaired. In these situations, psychiatric nurses can be more directive in the provision of services; and,
- Determination of alternative sources for consent when there is evidence that the patient is unable to consider the relevant issues of psychopharmacologic treatment. This may mean seeking judicial orders for treatment.

An additional feature of serving the best interests of the patient relates to the ethical obligation to develop and possess an understanding of issues related to patient confidentiality. Factors included in this dimension of obligation include the maintenance of confidentiality requirements in the following situations:

- In-person communication.
- Telephone requests for information.
- Inclusion of sensitive information in the clinical record. There are times when it is advisable to obtain patient consent prior to inclusion of sensitive information in the written document.
- Recognition of incidence of patient emergency when confidentiality and consent for release of information

may necessitate waiver if the best interests of the patient are to be served.

■ Separate personal working papers or a separate journal which is not a part of the clinical record and which may be used to record nursing activities associated with care of a patient as a log of events not typically entered in the patient record.

Contextual factors refer to the context of the situation—inclusive of providers, significant others, setting, social and financial considerations, and other influences which can affect the available options for care and treatment.

The nurse is ethically obligated to collaborate with patients, families, significant others, and health care providers to meet the needs of the patient and obtain optimal health care outcomes within the context of a given set of situational factors. An important implication of this obligation is that decisions regarding psychopharmacologic treatment be carried out in keeping with culture and other contextual issues.

The following expectations apply:

■ Obtain consent from the patient for collaboration in psychopharmacologic treatment and follow-up with identified family members, health care providers, community resources, and significant others;

■ Collaborate and lobby actively with community agencies, groups, and policy makers on behalf of the specialty populations who are the recipients of psychopharmacologic care; and,

■ Obtain and maintain a current knowledge and understanding of the state and federal laws and agency-specific responsibilities regarding advocacy for and referral of patients receiving psychopharmacologic care.

Two context-specific areas of psychiatric mental health nursing practice which require particular attention with regard to ethical and legal issues are research and negligence or malpractice.

Research

The psychiatric nurse has ethical obligations with regard to participation in psychopharmacological research activities. The obligations toward the patient include:

■ Assurance that the patient has received full disclosure regarding the research protocol, funding, and expected outcomes, including risks and benefits, as well as follow-up treatment.

■ Supporting the patient's decision to refuse either initial or continued participation in research projects.

■ Assurance of the patient's safety throughout the research study and upon discontinuation of the patient's participation, regardless of whether such discontinuation is initiated by the patient, is the decision of the investigators, or is the end of the study.

Nursing Actions

Nurses in psychiatric settings are ethically obligated to address inadequate, negligent, or illegal nursing and other patient care when standards of care for psychopharmacologic treatment have not been met. Expectations for addressing the perceived violation are dependent upon the education and the position of the individual nurse.

The following steps are options which could be taken by the nurse. They are listed by increasing levels of intervention.

■ Approach the individual care giver and determine whether there is a reasonable remedy for the concerns. The nurse must determine the appropriateness of supporting the care giver in achieving the remedy.

■ Document the issue and actions taken in the clinical record.

■ Bring the issue to the attention of the next level of nursing management as indicated or as required by institutional policy.

■ Report relevant information to the state board of nursing or other appropriate regulating body. This may be done anonymously, if necessary, to minimize risk for the nurse making the report.

The psychiatric mental health nurse has the ethical obligation to accept only patient assignments for which the nurse possesses sufficient knowledge, skill, and ability or has and uses available consultation. When this is not the case, the psychiatric mental health nurse has the ethical obligation to decline the assignment.

Conclusion

There was a consistency of opinion in this work group that the guidelines for psychopharmacology practice should include dimensions of ethical obligations for psychiatric mental health nurses. These obligations are regarded as the minimum for all nurses, regardless of level of preparation.

The reason for this approach rests in the notion that obligations should be viewed in a broad way, not dependent on level of training. Nonetheless, with additional education and independence of practice comes a higher level of ethical responsibility.

It should be noted that in the *Psychopharmacology Guidelines* presented in this book, there is not a specific section on legal/ethical issues. Rather, these issues have been integrated throughout. For further discussion of legal and ethical issues for psychiatric nurses, see the American Nurses Association *Statement on Psychiatric-Mental Health Clinical Nursing Practice and Standards on Psychiatric-Mental Health Clinical Nursing Practice* (American Nurses Association 1994).

PART II

AMERICAN NURSES ASSOCIATION

Psychopharmacology Guidelines for Psychiatric Mental Health Nurses

American Nurses Association

Psychopharmacology Guidelines for Psychiatric Mental Health Nurses

The contemporary practice of psychiatric mental health nursing is based on the integration and application of information from the biological, behavioral, social, and neurosciences. Each of these fields is expanding rapidly, requiring ongoing education to ensure incorporation of new findings into psychiatric mental health nursing practice.

This document describes the knowledge base psychiatric mental health nurses need in relation to one aspect of practice—psychopharmacology. It is intended only to inform and guide psychiatric mental health nursing education, practice, and research in this area. Thus, this document should not be considered part of any state's nurse practice act, or viewed as a requirement for licensure, or construed as a legal standard by which to judge psychiatric nursing practice.

These guidelines will be evaluated and updated regularly. Psychiatric mental health nurses will demonstrate expanding expertise in psychopharmacology based on the state of the science, education, experience, practice setting, patient needs, and professional goals.

I. Neurosciences

Commensurate with level of practice, the psychiatric mental health nurse integrates current knowledge from the neurosciences to understand etiological models, diagnostic issues, and treatment strategies for psychiatric illness.

Objectives

The psychiatric mental health nurse can:

- describe basic central nervous system structures and functions implicated in mental illness, such as the cerebrum, diencephalon, brain stem, basal ganglia, limbic system, and extrapyramidal motor system.
- describe basic mechanisms of neurotransmission at the synapse, such as neurochemical metabolism, role(s) of the pre- and post-synaptic membranes, re-uptake, receptor binding, and auto-regulation.
- describe the general functions of the major neurochemicals implicated in mental illness, such as serotonin, norepinephrine, dopamine, acetylcholine, GABA, and the peptides.
- describe the basic structure and function of the endocrine system, particularly as it is affected by the various hypothalamic-pituitary endocrine axes.

- identify the neurotransmitter system implicated in side-effect profiles of psychopharmacologic agents, such as blockade of cholinergic receptors (blurred vision, dry mouth, memory dysfunction), histaminic receptors (sedation, weight gain, hypotension), and adrenergic receptors (dizziness, postural hypotension, tachycardia).
- discuss the relevance of current biological hypotheses underlying major mental illnesses and the use of psychopharmacologic agents.
- demonstrate a familiarity with the increased lifetime risk of mental illness—for people who have a mentally ill first-degree (biological) relative—compared to the general population, based on genetic, epidemiologic, family, adoption, and twin research.
- describe normal sleep stages and identify circadian rhythm disturbances, such as decreased REM latency and phase shift disturbances as evidenced in psychiatric disorders.
- demonstrate familiarity with recent research findings from neuro-imaging techniques such as CT (computerized tomography), MRI (magnetic resonance imagining), PET (positron-emission tomography), and SPECT (single photon emission computerized tomography) as well as the psychiatric uses of these techniques.
- discuss the purposes and limitations of current biological tests used in the diagnosis and monitoring of mental illness.

II. Psychopharmacology

The psychiatric mental health nurse involved in the care of patients who have been prescribed psychopharmacologic agents demonstrates knowledge of psychopharmacologic principles—including pharmacokinetics, pharmacodynamics, drug classification, intended and unintended effects, and related nursing implications.

Objectives
The psychiatric mental health nurse can:

- describe psychopharmacologic agents based on the similarities and differences among drugs of the same and different classes.

- discuss the actions of psychopharmacologic agents that range from global human behavioral responses to those at a cellular level, such as the actions of lithium from mood stabilization to glomerular effects.
- differentiate the psychiatric symptoms targeted for psychopharmacologic intervention from medication side effects and toxicities, and the appropriate interventions to minimize each.
- apply basic principles of pharmacokinetics and pharmacodynamics, such as half-life, steady state, absorption, and metabolism, in general and as they relate to age, gender, race/ethnicity, and organ system function.
- identify the appropriate use of psychotherapeutic agents related to the psychiatric needs of special populations.
- involve patients and their families and significant others in the design and implementation of the medication treatment plan, taking into account patient readiness, knowledge, environment, beliefs and preferences, and lifestyle.
- identify factors that may prevent the active collaboration of patients with medication regimens, and strategies to minimize these risks.
- describe nonpsychopharmacologic interventions for target symptoms that are not responsive to psychopharmacologic interventions, psychiatric symptoms unlikely to respond to drug treatments, and drug side effects that are not treated with drugs.
- discuss the use of standardized rating scales for measuring symptom severity and clinical response to psychopharmacologic treatment, such as changes in target symptoms of illness and medication side effects.
- demonstrate the knowledge necessary to develop psychopharmacologic education and treatment plans based on current neurobiological concepts and the patient's lifestyle and recovery environment.

III. Clinical Management

The psychiatric mental health nurse applies principles from the neurosciences and psychopharmacology to provide safe and effective management of patients being treated with psychopharmacologic agents. Clinical management includes assessment, diagnosis, and treatment considerations.

A. ASSESSMENT

The psychiatric mental health nurse has the knowledge, skills, and ability to conduct and interpret patient assessments in relation to psychopharmacologic agents. Assessments include physical, neuropsychiatric, psychosocial, and psychopharmacologic parameters.

1. Physical Assessment

Objectives

The psychiatric mental health nurse can:

- collect health data related to past and present health problems and concurrent treatments for other psychiatric or medical problems the patient may have.
- collect health data related to current and past drug use (prescribed, over-the-counter, and illicit), current and past substance use (caffeine, nicotine, alcohol), and related health practices.
- conduct and/or interpret findings from a physical examination and laboratory studies to obtain information about pertinent organ system functioning.
- evaluate laboratory results that reflect drug effects on organ systems, drug blood levels and toxicities, and concurrent medical problems that may mimic or exacerbate psychiatric symptoms or drug effects.
- assess baseline and ongoing status of motor activity and sleep patterns, appetite, dietary practices and preferences, and functional status.

2. Neuropsychiatric Assessment

Objectives

The psychiatric mental health nurse can:

- conduct and/or interpret findings from a basic neuropsychiatric exam including gross cranial and peripheral nerve function; gait; muscle strength, function and range of motion; and mental status.
- identify chief neuropsychiatric complaints, presenting symptoms, and goals for psychopharmacologic interventions.
- make appropriate use of available informants and records to augment self-reports of neuropsychiatric assessment and premorbid patterns.
- demonstrate appropriate use of standardized rating scales to document mental status, drug effects on the core psychiatric symptomatology, and side effects such as those occurring in the extrapyramidal system.

3. Psychosocial Assessment

Objectives

The psychiatric mental health nurse can:

- utilize demographic and personal information for the development of a patient-centered medication treatment plan, considering the patient's ethnic/cultural background, developmental stage, cognitive ability, educational level, reading level and comprehension, socioeconomic status, and capacity to ask questions and seek answers.
- assess the effects of psychopharmacologic interventions on the patient's quality of life, including the impact on interpersonal relationships, appearance, work and leisure functioning, diet, sleep, sexual performance, family planning, functional status, financial status, self-esteem, and perception of stigma associated with medication intervention.
- identify actual and potential sources of support for the patient such as significant others; household and family members; friendships and informal relationships; work relationships; and affiliations with community, social, and religious organizations.
- identify actual and potential barriers to treatment within the patient and the environment, such as impaired functional status, cultural/ethnic/religious beliefs and practices, absence of a support system, limited cognitive abilities, stressors, financial hardships, deficient coping skills, impaired capacity to collaborate with treatment, limited transportation, and patient and family perceptions of illness and medication treatment.

4. Psychopharmacological Assessment

Objectives

The psychiatric mental health nurse can:

- identify patient-related variables pertinent to the risk/benefit assessment of psychopharmacologic treatment such as demographic (age, gender, ethnicity/race); physical (organ system function, concurrent illnesses); treatment (concurrent treatments); and personal (past history, self-care practices, goals for treatment, ability to pay, and quality of life) characteristics.
- identify drug-related variables important in the risk/benefit assessment of psychopharmacologic agents, such as safety and efficacy, advantages and disadvan-

tages compared to other drugs in the same class, therapeutic range, side-effect profile, toxicities, contraindications, potential interactions with other drugs or diet, polypharmacy considerations, safety in overdose, availability of information on long-term side effects, and cost.

- evaluate the appropriateness and least restrictive nature of psychopharmacologic interventions for each patient.
- assess the ability and willingness of the patient and significant others to give informed consent for treatment with psychopharmacologic agents.
- utilize standardized behavioral rating scales to assess and monitor drug effects and changes in target symptoms.

B. DIAGNOSIS

The psychiatric mental health nurse has the knowledge, skills, and ability to utilize appropriate nursing, psychiatric, and medical diagnostic classification systems to guide psychopharmacologic management of patients with mental illness.

Objectives
The psychiatric mental health nurse can:

- utilize standardized diagnostic systems as appropriate for making nursing (North American Nursing Diagnostic Association-NANDA or other nursing systems) and psychiatric diagnoses (*Diagnostic and Statistical Manual—DSM*), and interpreting medical diagnoses (*International Classification of Diseases—ICD*).
- elicit information—from the patient and other appropriate informants or records—that is relevant to the diagnostic process.
- make nursing diagnostic judgments that include information about but are not limited to the psychiatric diagnosis, symptoms targeted for psychopharmacologic intervention, clinical diagnoses, physical symptoms, coping responses, functional status, developmental level, learning capabilities, and the patient's quality of life and preferences.
- use these diagnostic judgments as the basis for setting treatment priorities and selecting and assessing nursing interventions, including management of psychopharmacologic agents.
- communicate and integrate diagnostic impressions

with other members of the health care team. This can include representatives of managed care enterprises.

C. TREATMENT

The psychiatric mental health nurse takes an active role in the treatment of patients with mental illness and integrates prescribed psychopharmacologic interventions into a cohesive, multidimensional plan of care.

1. Initiation

Objectives
The psychiatric mental health nurse can:

- use information obtained during the nursing assessment to develop a medication treatment plan that considers target symptoms, side effects, concurrent treatments and health status, requirements of specific drugs, dietary and activity considerations, and patient-related variables.
- demonstrate an understanding of pharmacokinetic and pharmacodynamic principles that underlie safe and effective psychopharmacologic management, such as how dosing and tapering schedules are adjusted, and how patient-related variables are integrated.
- relate the length of time it may take a drug to have a therapeutic effect, the time it takes for expected side effects to occur and remit, early signs of unexpected or adverse events, and nursing interventions to reduce side effects and facilitate therapeutic response.
- apply principles of health education and nursing ethics and legal parameters in informing patients about medication treatments, risks/benefits, concurrent and alternative treatments, and informed consent.
- apply least restrictive principles and advance directives to avoid the overuse or under-use of medications as chemical restraints, and to anticipate safety needs, such as potential for harm to self or others, suicidality, aggression, assaultiveness, and violence.

2. Stabilization

Objectives
The psychiatric mental health nurse can:

- monitor target symptoms, acute medication effects, and functional status throughout the course of treatment.

- utilize information obtained from therapeutic drug monitoring, laboratory values, standardized rating scales, and patient and family reports to monitor progress.
- recognize indications for modifying dosing schedules and describe alternative medication strategies as needed.

3. Maintenance

Objectives

The psychiatric mental health nurse can:

- develop a plan of care—in collaboration with the patient, family, and other care providers as appropriate— which includes monitoring outcomes such as efficacy of treatment, changes in target symptoms, emergence of long-term side effects, laboratory values and physical findings relevant to specific medications, and occurrence of destabilizing stressors.
- identify possible barriers to maintenance care, such as issues regarding transportation, finances, birth control, child care, support system, relocation, cultural/ ethnic differences, therapeutic relationship, and psychosocial stressors; and, the patient's understanding of symptom reduction, symptom exacerbation, and side effects.
- facilitate the patient's transition from one treatment setting to another, such as from the hospital to the community, from one care provider to another, and from one treatment to another.
- develop a patient-education program for relapse prevention that can include self-monitoring techniques and teaching tools such as medication cards, handouts, diaries, bibliographies, and other materials to enhance ongoing education of patients, families, and significant others.
- enhance health promotion with restoration techniques that can be individualized for the patient and integrated with medication treatments, such as diet; exercise; leisure activities; and community, social and religious affiliations.
- assist the patient, family, and significant others to establish advance directives regarding emergency inter-

ventions, including the use of psychopharmacologic agents.

4. Discontinuation and Follow-Up

Objectives

The psychiatric mental health nurse can:

- relate current recommended practices regarding psychopharmacologic maintenance requirements and duration of treatment for specific psychiatric disorders.
- discuss issues related to discontinuation of medication, including tapering schedules, and potential sequelae, such as withdrawal, dependence, rebound effects, and return of symptoms of illness.
- develop with the patient, family, and significant others a plan for self-care in a post-medication phase that considers assessments of quality of life, predisposing stressors, re-emergence of symptoms, appropriate use of support systems, and contact sources for potential re-evaluation of treatment status.
- assess the patient before, during, and after the course of treatment, clearly differentiating between changes in the patient as a result of illness effects, drug effects, premorbid personality characteristics, effects of aging, and effects of the environment.

IV. Recommendations

These *Guidelines* are designed to be used as a tool for psychiatric mental health nurses to determine their knowledge and skill in psychopharmacology and to design a plan for their continued growth in this field. The *Guidelines* can also be used as the basis for the development of curricula and continuing education programs for psychiatric mental health nurses in psychopharmacology. New information in this field should be added to the *Guidelines* on a regular basis.

As a set of guidelines, this document should not be used in legal proceedings or as an evaluation of nurses' competence in this field by institutions or state or federal agencies.

Summary and Recommendations

Michele T. Laraia, R.N., M.S.N.
Sarah R. Stanley, M.S., R.N.

This summary of the findings from the Psychopharmacology Project reflects two years of work and the efforts of many individuals. Hopefully, the recommendations will provide a basis for the increased integration of psychopharmacology content into the formal and informal educational programs of nurses, as well as the fuller application of this information in quality nursing care provided to persons with mental illness and their families.

One initiative of the Psychopharmacology Project was an evaluation of the psychiatric mental health nursing environment related to psychopharmacology. This environmental review included: education, publications (textbooks, journals, computer programs, and videos), and conferences. This review proved useful in documenting what is currently provided within the specialty for psychiatric mental health nurses related to psychopharmacology.

In addition, the practice setting environment for psychiatric mental health nurses was reviewed. A National Conference on Competencies in Psychopharmacology for Psychiatric Nurses provided a thorough review of what psychiatric mental health nurses need in the practice setting, related to psychopharmacology and related neurosciences, as articulated by leaders in the field. From the perspective of both clinicians and educators across the country, there is a great and immediate need for information and guidelines by which nurses can pursue ongoing knowledge in the fields of psychopharmacology and related neurosciences.

The national psychopharmacology conference included several representatives of consumer advocacy groups for persons with mental illness. Not surprisingly, consumer groups are also challenging mental health professionals to reconsider exclusively psychodynamic explanations of mental illness. This is in light of recent developments in the neurosciences, particularly those involving genetics, the results of neuro-imaging techniques, and the effects of psychopharmacologic agents. These groups believe that the individuals and families they represent have long felt blamed for causing mental illness in their family members.

To ensure that psychiatric mental health nurses are prepared to assimilate and communicate the explosion of critical scientific information in this field, it is essential that a number of changes be made. A rapid step forward in almost all of the areas reviewed is recommended so that psychiatric mental health nurses can continue to turn to their specialty for the information necessary to care for psychiatric patients, teach psychiatric mental health nursing, and conduct research in the specialty.

The number of nurses entering graduate programs in psychiatric nursing has declined over the past two decades. In addition, less than 20 percent of master's-prepared nurses are under 35 years of age (NIMH 1990). Younger nurses are not joining the ranks of psychiatric nursing. The loss of federal funding for graduate education in nursing has played a major role in this decline.

To garner support and attract new students to psychiatric mental health nursing and graduate study in the field, both undergraduate and graduate curricula must keep pace with the developments in the field of mental health, including the neurosciences and psychopharmacology. Failure to do so carries the risk of continuing the decline in the number of psychiatric mental health nurses prepared to practice in this country at a time when the need for mental health professionals has never been greater.

Specifically, undergraduate- and graduate-level nursing programs must include comprehensive and current information about the neurosciences and psychopharmacology as they relate to mental illness. Undergraduate nursing programs should provide a solid foundation in neuroscience and psychopharmacology, while graduate programs in psychiatric mental health nursing should require advanced learning, clinical application, and research inquiry in these essential fields.

As more is learned about the genetic, developmental, and environmental determinants of mental illness, treatment is likely to become increasingly multimodal and multidisciplinary (Institute of Medicine 1989). Therefore, psychiatric nurse clinicians and specialists will need education that extends beyond the traditional modalities of individual, family, and group psychotherapy (Krauss 1993).

Given the proliferation of physiological tests, psychopharmacologic agents, and other somatic treatments, added educational effort in this area is essential. Closely related clinical skills, such as physical assessment, medication management, and the use of valid and reliable methods of monitoring drug response are equally important. Mastering this content and articulating the roles of psychiatric mental health nurses in these rapidly expanding areas will offer exciting career opportunities for nurses entering the specialty, while access to mental health services and the quality of care provided patients with psychiatric illness will be improved.

While psychiatric nursing publications have shown an increased focus on psychopharmacology and the neurosciences over the past few years, they need additional content to provide nurses with current, comprehensive information in these rapidly changing fields. These publications have a wide readership and can make an important contribution to continuing education in this area, but it is not clear at present whether editors and authors view the fields of neurosciences, including psychopharmacology, as essential areas of psychiatric nursing practice.

Furthermore, in this age of expanding automated services, psychiatric mental health nurses must be better able to access information in an automated format. Changes need to be made to facilitate nurses' computerized searches of databases related to journal articles and computer-assisted learning programs. These technologies must be utilized in today's rapidly changing health care environment so the profession can keep up with critical information necessary to provide excellence in patient care, based upon the integration of new theories, interventions, and research findings.

Psychiatric nursing conferences are a resource to the field in their presentation and dissemination of information about psychopharmacology and related neurosciences to nurse clinicians and specialists. The number of pre-conference workshops and conference presentations in these areas has been increasing over the past few years and almost every major psychiatric nursing conference program now includes these topics, indicating the high nurse-consumer demand for this information. Funding for conferences offering this information, as well as scholarships for those attending these conferences, should be made available to continue to support this important learning resource in this age of dwindling health care training and education funds.

The *Psychopharmacology Guidelines for Psychiatric Mental Health Nurses* are the definitive outcome of the Psychopharmacology Project. The *Guidelines* should be disseminated to all psychiatric mental health nurses, every institution in which nurses are educated, and each practice setting where patients receive care.

They should be used as guides to direct changes in the way psychiatric mental health nurses view their roles in the care of the mentally ill, in the advocacy for mentally ill patients and their families, in the education of psychiatric nurses, in the research of evolving areas of practice, and in interdisciplinary collaboration with other professionals in the health care field.

The ANA Task Force on Psychopharmacology therefore proposes that NIMH and ANA call for a national initiative to support the knowledge base and role of psychiatric mental health nurses in the administration, health education, and therapeutic maintenance of patients receiving psychopharmacologic medications. The future should include the refinement of levels of psychopharmacology practice by psychiatric mental health nurses, including the appropriate credentialing of psychiatric mental health nurses in psychopharmacology.

In addition, training grants for nursing programs—particularly at the graduate level—that demonstrate contemporary course work in psychopharmacology and related neurosciences should be made available to attract promising students to the specialty and to support them. Grant money for fellowships for pre-doctoral nurses in these fields will greatly enhance the treatment and research components of the specialty of psychiatric mental health nursing. Post-doctoral fellowships should be offered to nurses working in these fields at salaries commensurate with their experience and education.

Because of the rapid and comprehensive changes—

related to psychopharmacology—needed in the nursing environment, continuing education programs in the neurosciences and psychopharmacology should be supported, continuously updated, and made available to all psychiatric mental health nurses.

Equally important, legislation and regulations should allow patients access to psychiatric mental health nurses as primary mental health care providers; allow reimbursement to them for the services they provide; and reduce unnecessary federal and state restrictions on their practice. Finally, at every level, government and private agencies should include psychiatric nurses on regulatory and decision-making panels and commissions regarding mental health diagnosis, treatment, and service delivery issues.

This is a time of unprecedented change and opportunity within the health and mental health care fields. The specialty of psychiatric mental health nursing and the profession of nursing as a whole, will be greatly affected by every initiative and strategy that is developed as a result of the findings of the Psychopharmacology Project and the *Psychopharmacology Guidelines for Psychiatric Mental Health Nurses*. Most of all, the responsibility for action lies with the individual nurse and with psychiatric mental health nurses as a group to keep abreast of knowledge in their field and apply it on a daily basis in the care of patients with mental illness and their families.

Bibliography

American Nurses Association. 1985. *Code for nurses with interpretive statements.* Kansas City, MO: the Author.

American Nurses Association. 1994. *A statement on psychiatric-mental health clinical nursing practice and standards on psychiatric-mental health clinical nursing practice.* Washington, DC: the Author.

American Psychiatric Association. 1994. *Diagnostic and statistical manual (DSM).* Washington, DC: the Author.

Finke, L.M., DeLeon Siantz, M.L. 1992. *Collaboration for improvement of practice with severely mentally and emotionally disturbed children and adolescents.* Washington, DC: NIMH, Division of Clinical Research Education and Training Branch.

Institute of Medicine. 1989. *Research on children and adolescents with mental, behavioral and developmental disorders: Mobilizing a national initiative.* Washington, DC: National Academy Press.

Jonsen, A.R., Siegler, M., and Winslade, W.J. 1992. *Clinical ethics: A practical approach to ethical decisions in clinical medicine.* New York: McGraw Hill.

Karaffa, M., ed. 1993. *International classification of disease*, 9th revision. Los Angeles: Practice Management Information Corporation.

Krauss, J.B. 1993. *Health care reform: Essential mental health services.* Washington, DC: American Nurses Publishing.

National Adivsory Council. 1992. Report to Congress on healthcare reform. Washington, DC: National Institute of Mental Health. April, 1993.

National Institute of Mental Health. 1990. *Mental health, United States, 1990.* Eds. R.W. Manderscheid and M.A. Sonnenschein. DHHS Publication Number (ADM) 90-1708. Washington, DC: DHHS.

North American Nursing Diagnosis Association. 1992. NANDA nursing diagnoses: Definitions and classifications 1992-1993. Philadelphia: the Author.

APPENDICES

ANA National Psychopharmacology Conference Participant List

Members of the ANA Psychopharmacology Task Force

Michele T. Laraia, R.N., M.S.N., Chair
Division of Psychiatric Nursing
Department of Psychiatry and
   Behavioral Sciences
Medical University of South Carolina
Charleston, SC 43925

Linda S. Beeber, Ph.D., R.N.
Syracuse University
College of Nursing, 13078
Syracuse, NY 13244-3290

Gloria B. Callwood, Ph.D., R.N.
Psychiatric Nurse Consultant
   Coordinator
Nursing Department QA&I Program
St. Thomas Hospital
St. Thomas, USVI 00802

Susan Caverly, M.A., R.N.
2425 214th Place, S.W.
Brier, WA 98036

Jeanne Anne Clement, Ed.D., R.N.
The Ohio State University
College of Nursing
1585 Neil Avenue
Columbus, OH 43210

Faye Gary, Ed.D., R.N.
Box 100187
Gainesville, FL 32610

Norman L. Keltner, Ed.D., R.N.
University of Alabama, Birmingham
University Station
Birmingham, AL 35294

Mary Ann Nihart, M.A., R.N.
Private Practice, Turning Point
   Center, SF
Consultant & Partner, Professional
   Growth Facilitators
San Clemente, California
Clinical Nurse Specialist, VA,
   Menlo Park, California
146 Hilton Lane
Pacifica, CA 94044

Lawrence Scahill, R.N., M.S.N., M.P.H.
Yale School of Nursing, Yale Child
   Study Center
230 S. Frontage Road
New Haven, CT 06517

Susan Simmons-Alling, M.S.N., R.N.
1204 Pond Road
Spring Lake Heights, NJ 07762

Sarah R. Stanley, M.S., R.N., C.N.A., C.S.
Senior Policy Analyst
Department of Practice, Economics,
   and Policy
600 Maryland Avenue, SW
Suite 100 West
Washington, DC 20024-2571

Sandra Talley, M.N., R.N., A.N.P.
University of Utah
25 So. Medical Drive
Salt Lake City, UT 84103

ANA Staff

Winifred Carson, Esquire
Senior Policy Fellow, Legal Affairs
Department of Practice, Economics,
   and Policy

Valarie Carty
Administrative Assistant
Department of Practice, Economics,
   and Policy

CMHS Project Officer

Carol Bush, Ph.D., R.N.
Acting Chief, Human Resources
   Development and Planning Branch
Center for Mental Health Services
   Room 7C-02
5600 Fisher's Lane
Rockville, MD 20857

Consultant

Karen Soeken, Ph.D.
University of Maryland
15702 Tasa Place
Laurel, MD 20707

Conference Participants Selected by Their State Nurses Associations

Beth Abeth-Moore, M.S., R.N.
1853 Oyster Bay Lane
Suffolk, VA 23436

Carolyn Billings, M.S.N., R.N., C.S.
3410 Hillsborough Street
Raleigh, NC 27607

Elizabeth C. Blackstead, M.N., R.N., C.S.
1015 Brookside Avenue
Redlands, CA 92373

Mary Ann Boyd, Ph.D. D.N.S., R.N., C.S.
233 Oak Tree Drive
Columbia, IL 62236

Deborah Ann Pariso Brown, M.S., R.N.
601 Montcalm Place
St. Paul, MN 55116

Mary Ann Camann, R.N., M.N., C.S.
Kennesaw State College
Department of Nursing, P.O. Box 444
Marietta, GA 30061

Karen Babich, Ph.D., R.N.
520 Dartmouth Avenue
Silver Spring, MD 20910

Andrea C. Bostrom, Ph.D., R.N.
2501 Crest Drive
Kalamazoo, MI 49008

Colleen Brill, M.S., R.N.
Weber State University
Nursing Program
Ogden, UT 84408-3903

Frances A. Brown, M.S.E.D., R.N., C.S.
7700 Parakeet Avenue
Las Vegas, NV 89128

Corinne L. Conlon, M.S., R.N.
3 Omega Court
Barboursville, VA 22923

Jamie Cook, Ph.D., R.N.
1514 South Magnolia Drive
Tallahassee, FL 32301

Carmel Dato, M.S., R.N., C.S.
54 West 16th Street #4J
New York, NY 10011

Billinda K. Dubbert, M.S., R.N.
12338 Field Lark Court
Fairfax, VA 22033

Janice Cooke Feigenbaum, Ph.D., R.N.
8 Argosy Drive
Amherst, NY 14226

Anne H. Fishel, Ph.D., M.S.N.
University of North Carolina
School of Nursing
C.B. 7460 Carrington Hall
Chapel Hill, NC 27599-7460

Carol A. Glod, M.S., R.N., C.S.
300 South Road
Bedford, MA 01730

Patricia Grimm, Ph.D., M.S.N., R.N.
The John Hopkins University
School of Nursing
600 N. Wolfe Street
Baltimore, MD 21287-1316

Bonnie Hagerty, Ph.D., R.N.
University of Michigan
2352 NIB School of Nursing
Ann Arbor, MI 48109

Joanne D. Joyner, M.S.N., R.N., C.S.
4905 Blagden Terrace, NW
Washington, DC 20011

Mary Kunes-Connell, Ph.D., R.N.
2315 South 47th Street
Omaha, NE 68106

Marilee Namba Kauhi, M.S., R.N.
891 Hoomaemae Street
Pearl City, HI 96782

Barbara J. Limandri, D.N.Sc., R.N., C.S.
Oregon Health Sciences University
School of Nursing
Department of Mental Health Nursing
  SNMHN
3181 SW Sam Jackson Park Road
Portland, OR 97201-3098

Patti Leger, M.S.N., R.N.
Children's Bellevue
400 112th Avenue, NE, Suite 110
Bellevue, WA 98004

Geoffry McEnany, M.S., R.N.
6745 Sobrante Road
Oakland, CA 94611

Bruce P. Mericle, M.S., R.N.
420 Sanhican Drive
Trenton, NJ 08618-5017

Elizabeth F. Mitchell, M.S.N., R.N.
444 Delwiche Drive
Green Bay, WI 54302

Marian Newton, Ph.D., R.N., M.S.N.
33 Jefferson Road
Glenmont, NY 12077

Margaret F. Raynor, M.S.E.D., R.N.
Staff Development Director
Dorothea Dix Hospital
703 Palmer Drive
Raleigh, NC 27603

Shirley Spencer, R.N.
P.O. Box 10
Lee's Summit, MO 64063

Maryellen McBride, M.N., A.R.N.P.,
  C.N.S.
1700 College
Topeka, KS 66621

Anne Roe Mealey, Ph.D., M.S.E.D., R.N.
W 2917 Ft. George Wright Drive
Spokane, WA 99204

Rebecca A. Michaels, M.S.N., R.N.
Macon College
100 College Station Drive
Macon, GA 31297

Noreen M. Nowak, M.S.N., R.N., C.S.
St. Francis Hospital Center
Mental Health Services
Beech Grove, IN 46107

Teresa Peduzzi, R.N.
10122 Farmington Drive
Fairfax, VA 22030

Bonnie Selzler, M.S.N., R.N.
1664 Witchita Drive
Bismarck, ND 58504

Gail W. Stuart, Ph.D., R.N., F.A.A.N.
Division of Psychiatric Nursing
Department of Psychiatry, MUSC
171 Ashley Avenue
Charleston, SC 29439

Rosalyn B. Tolbert, Ph.D., R.N., M.S.N.
UTA School of Nursing
P.O. Box 19407
Arlington, TX 76019

Margaret S. Wacker, Ph.D., R.N., C.S.
876 Plainfield Pike
North Scituate, RI 02857

Evelyn K. Tomes, Ph.D., R.N., M.S.N.
College of Nursing
Howard University
Washington, DC 20059

Louise C. Waszak, Ph.D., R.N.
West Virginia University
School of Nursing
3027 HSCN Box 9620
Morgantown, WV 26506-9620

American Nurses Association

600 Maryland Avenue SW, Suite 100 West, Washington, DC 20024-2571
202-554-4444 • Fax: 202-554-2262

Virginia Trotter Betts, JD, MSN, RN
President

Barbara K. Redman, PhD, RN, FAAN
Executive Director

October 6, 1992

Dear Dean,

Please find enclosed a very important document—a survey designed by the American Nurses Association Council on Psychiatric and Mental Health Nursing's **Task Force on Psychopharmacology** for a project funded by the National Institute of Mental Health. This task force is charged to carry out several activities with the ultimate goal of improving the care of the mentally ill in this country. In keeping with this charge, the task force will assess nursing curricula, publications, and conferences regarding nursing psychopharmacology content, and conduct a workshop in March 1993 to develop standards on core competencies for psychiatric nurses in psychopharmacology.

Your school is being asked to participate in this project and support the speciality of psychiatric and mental health nursing in reaching these goals. The enclosed survey will enable us to assess psychopharmacology content currently being taught in schools of nursing. The survey has been designed with the participant in mind, and we hope you will find it clear and concise.

Please ask the most appropriate person on your nursing faculty **GRADUATE PROGRAM** to complete this survey and return it in the enclosed business reply envelope to the ANA by October 26, 1992. The return of the survey will indicate your agreement to participate. All information will be reported as aggregate data, and the names of schools and faculty will be held in strict confidence.

You may call Michele Laraia, MSN, RN, Chair, ANA Psychopharmacology Task Force, directly at the Medical University of South Carolina (803-792-7935), or Sarah Stanley at ANA headquarters (202-554-4444, ext. 289), if you have any questions regarding the survey or this project. The results of the survey, as well as the entire project, will be available by Fall 1993, and you should indicate on the survey form if you wish to have the survey results sent to you. Thank you for facilitating this important work.

Sincerely,

Virginia Trotter Betts

Virginia Trotter Betts, JD, MSN, RN
President, American Nurses Association

Enclosures

Excerpts from the Keynote Address

Efficacy of Major Psychotropic Medications: Critical Role for Psychiatric Nursing

Jeanne Fox, Ph.D., R.N., F.A.A.N.

The effective care and treatment of individuals with psychiatric disorders is of concern for all psychiatric nurses. The following pages contain excerpts from the keynote address to the Psychopharmacology Practice Conference, March 1993. This address reviewed what is known about the efficacy of psychopharmacologic and psychosocial treatments for individuals suffering from major mental illness, although the focus of this brief report will be on psychopharmacologic interventions. The information contained herein was taken directly from background papers prepared for the National Mental Health Advisory Council report to the U.S. Congress, submitted in April 1993. The full report is available to the public and the reader is encouraged to obtain it. This report should be referenced and credited for any information used in the following condensed report.

Treatments for Schizophrenia

The accumulated evidence regarding currently available medications for the treatment of schizophrenia is impressive—they serve both to treat the acute symptoms of schizophrenia and to prevent or delay relapse. Some studies suggest that guaranteeing medication compliance through the use of injectable medication can reduce the risk of relapse, but some schizophrenic patients will experience return of symptoms even when medication receipt is guaranteed.

A substantial body of literature addresses the feasibility and potential benefits of reducing the amount of medication received during long-term maintenance treatment in order to minimize side effects and enhance community functioning. Continuous low-dosage administration is associated with increased risk of relapse or minor episodes. The time required for episode to develop depends on the dosage level. However, lower dosage is also associated with reduced side effects, improved social functioning for patients who do not relapse, and in at least one study, reduced manifestation of the abnormal movements of tardive dyskinesia.

One strategy—targeted or intermittent treatment—has been associated with substantially increased rates of relapse compared to more standard doses of medication and there is little evidence that symptom reduction or social functioning improves results. This may be a treatment strategy to be considered for patients who refuse medication but who will remain in contact with a treatment team. There is some evidence that relapse rates are lower with early, targeted treatment than with later crisis intervention.

Among the newer medications reviewed at this time, clozapine is the most exciting. Because of its risk of agranulocytosis, use of clozapine is restricted to treatment of nonresponsive or neuroleptic-intolerant patients. Clozapine's effectiveness in this difficult to treat population is impressive. However, there are no long-term comparative trials with this drug or studies that have examined either maintenance dosing strategies or the question of relapse among patients who initially respond to clozapine.

Another new dopamine-serotonin antagonist which looks very promising, risperidone, showed equal efficacy to clozapine when used in low doses and improvement in both positive and negative symptoms of schizophrenia without increased EPS when compared to haloperidol. The advantage of risperidone over clozapine is that it does not require frequent blood monitoring.

A new generation of antipsychotic agents that will become widely available during the next few years is anticipated. Although results from clinical trials with these agents are still limited, the role of these and other similar drugs that are likely to be developed will be considerable in the future.

Care and treatment for schizophrenia extend beyond pharmacologic interventions. Among the most important questions to be answered in the treatment of schizophrenia are those that involve the relationships of pharmacologic and psychosocial treatments, particularly individual psychotherapeutic approaches, group psychotherapy, and family therapies. The few studies to date provide compelling evidence for the continuation of inquiry in this important area.

Treatments for Bipolar Disorders

At least 80 percent of patients who have an initial episode of mania will have one or more subsequent episodes. Because recurring episodes have a cumulative deteriorative effect on functioning and treatment response, the sooner bipolar patients are diagnosed and treated, the better their chances are for recovery.

For treatment purposes, bipolar disorder is divided into three stages: acute mania, acute depression, and maintenance. Lithium is the standard treatment for acute mania, and its effectiveness is solidly supported by experimental evidence. The anticonvulsant drugs carbamazepine and valproate have been shown to be comparable to lithium and superior to placebo in treating acute mania. ECT, another effective biologic treatment for acute mania, is a valuable option for several groups of bipolar patients: 1) pregnant women who cannot take lithium; 2) patients who are unresponsive to drug therapy; 3) severely manic patients; and 4) patients in mixed states who have a high risk of suicide.

Acute bipolar depression has been successfully treated with a number of agents, including monoamine oxidase inhibitors, lithium, tricyclic antidepressants, and second-generation antidepressants (e.g., bupropion). Other biologic approaches such as ECT, sleep deprivation, and light therapy have been effective as supplemental therapy in many patients.

For maintenance therapy, lithium is again the drug of choice. Carbamazepine and valproate are effective as alternatives or adjuncts to lithium therapy. The tricyclic antidepressant imipramine has been found to be less effective than lithium in preventing manic episodes but equally as effective in preventing depressive episodes. Bupropion and verapamil have also shown success in preliminary trials.

Other drugs are currently being investigated for their possible roles in treating patients with bipolar disorder. Some of the most promising are calcium channel blockers, including verapamil and nimodipine.

Treatments for Major Depression

Antidepressant medications have been shown to treat effectively all forms of major depressive disorder (MDD). Barring contraindications to these agents, antidepressant medications are first-line treatments for MDD when: 1) the depression is severe; 2) there are psychotic features (the addition of an antipsychotic is required for maximum efficacy); 3) there are melancholic or atypical symptom features (the MAOIs are especially effective); 4) the patient prefers medication; 5) psychotherapy by a competent trained therapist is not available; 6) the patient has shown a prior positive response to medication; or 7) prophylactic maintenance treatment is indicated.

The typical first drugs of choice include the secondary amine tricyclics (nortriptyline, desipramine), as well as the newer agents (bupropion, fluoxetine, and sertraline). In general, these drugs have equal efficacy but fewer side effects than the parent tertiary amines. Thus, they are also preferred in the elderly. The second choice drugs are often utilized as alternative agents for patients with special pre-

sentations or needs. These include the tertiary amine tricyclics (amitriptyline, imipramine), trazodone, the MAOIs, and selected anxiolytic medications.

While no one antidepressant is clearly more effective than another, the selection of drug depends on a variety of factors: short- and long-term side effects; prior positive/negative response; first-degree relatives responding to a medication; age; concurrent medical illnesses; compliance history; type of depression; once-a-day dosing availability; lifestyle considerations; cost of the medication; the practitioner's experience with the agent; and patient and family preference.

Long-term side effects must be considered, especially if the patient is a candidate for maintenance therapy. It should be noted, however, that many side effects abate with long-term treatment. The newer antidepressants (bupropion, fluoxetine, sertraline, trazodone) are associated with fewer long-term side effects, such as weight gain, than the older tricyclic medications.

Some evidence suggests a lower response to the use of tricyclics alone when the following conditions are present: 1) atypical symptom features; 2) psychotic features; 3) depressions complicated by personality disorder; and 4) severe melancholic depressions in the elderly. It has also been shown that when medication is stopped, the rate of long-term wellness is drastically reduced. A study conducted by NIMH (1985) found that patients with three or more episodes of MDD have a 90 percent chance of a fourth episode. Several studies have suggested that antidepressant medications are successful in preventing recurrent episodes in patients with histories of depression.

To date there are no well-established predictors regarding which patients are likely to benefit from combination treatment using medications and nonpharmacologic interventions. Choosing to enhance one type of treatment with another therapeutic approach appears to be a challenge each clinician must deal with by utilizing the progress of the patient and augmenting treatment in the areas most needed.

Panic Disorder: Efficacy of Current Treatments

Available evidence documents that at least 75 percent of patients will have a good response to tricyclic antidepressants, monoamine oxidase inhibitors, and benzodiazepines, which are all approximately equal in efficacy and side effects. Medications may be even more effective when combined with cognitive and behavioral techniques.

Tricyclics and newer agents: Imipramine, the most frequently and extensively studied of the tricyclic antidepressants, has had consistently excellent results. It generally requires four to six weeks or longer before significant clinical improvement is achieved. Other antidepressants with demonstrated utility for panic disorder include clomipramine, fluvoxamine, maprotiline, nortriptyline, amitriptyline, doxepin, fluoxetine, and paroxetine.

Monoamine oxidase inhibitors: Although the monoamine oxidase inhibitors have been somewhat less extensively studied, they have been shown to be comparable to the tricyclic antidepressants in the treatment of panic disorder.

Benzodiazepines: Alprazolam, the most studied of the benzodiazepines in the treatment of panic disorder, has comparable efficacy to the tricyclic antidepressants and monoamine oxidase inhibitors. The principal advantages to using alprazolam include: achieves clinical improvement rapidly; is effective in the first week of treatment, and is well tolerated by most patients. The greatest disadvantage for the benzodiazepines is that some patients experience a withdrawal syndrome when they are discontinued, though this can be minimized if the medicine is tapered slowly, gradually, and flexibly, and if the patient is prepared for the possible transient recurrence of some panic symptoms.

Probably the most frequently employed strategy by clinicians is to begin a benzodiazepine and an antidepressant simultaneously to take advantage of the rapid onset of efficacy with the benzodiazepine. Although this strategy has not been studied extensively, it appears to be effective and reasonable.

Length of treatment: Most patients are treated for 12 to 18 months and medications are then slowly tapered over at least 4 to 12 weeks. Although 35 percent to 45 percent do well after medication discontinuation, relapse is frequent and treatment may need to be reinstated. Longer periods of treatment (18 months versus 6 months) appear to reduce relapse rates.

Combined treatments: The most effective treatment for panic disorder is a combination of behavioral techniques and medication, though definitive evidence to support this position is limited. Several trials are underway which should provide definitive evidence concerning the potential value of combined treatment.

Obsessive-Compulsive Disorders: Efficacy of Treatments

Pharmacotherapy of OCD: In a variety of studies, 85 percent of patients on clomipramine demonstrated some improvement while fewer than 5 percent of those on placebo improved. Approximately 60 percent of the subjects who received clomipramine improved at least moderately. In addition, there are a number of studies that compared at least two drugs head to head without a placebo. Clomipramine and other serotonin re-uptake inhibitors (SSRIs) have often been compared in a controlled manner to other agents. In each of these cases, the SSRIs (clomipramine, fluvoxamine, fluoxetine, and sertraline) were significantly better than other agents. Several controlled trials have compared two SSRIs and failed to show any significant difference between them in terms of efficacy (in part, this may be due to low numbers of subjects enrolled in these studies).

Combined treatments: Currently, antidepressant medications are routinely used in combination with behavior therapy and with anecdotal evidence indicating this to be an efficient treatment approach. However, the literature contains only two comparisons of behavior therapy versus clomipramine, with only one testing the interaction of the two. Clomipramine has also been used in reports of childhood OCD in combination with behavior therapy. Good results have been obtained but the unique contributions of these treatments and their interaction await further controlled study.

Thus, there is overwhelming evidence that specific pharmacologic agents are effective in lessening symptoms of OCD in many patients. The combination of both pharmacotherapy and behavioral treatment optimizes the individual patient's potential for recovery and the majority of patients can now expect to lead relatively normal lives, to work, and to function well in families and in social situations.

Summary

Considerable information is available about the efficacy of psychopharmacologic, psychotherapeutic, and combined therapies and interventions for persons with mental illnesses. This information is essential for generalist and advanced practice psychiatric nurses and should be available to all health service providers in primary care as well as mental health specialty delivery sites. Advanced practice psychiatric nurses should play a pivotal role in the dissemination and updating of this knowledge in local practice communities.

From: National Institute of Mental Health Advisory Council Report to Congress April 1993. Washington, DC: the Author.

Consumer Panel Presentation

Persons Experiencing the Effects of Mental Disorders: What Psychiatric Nurses Need to Know about Medication Management: the Family Perspective

Evelyn McElroy, Ph.D., R.N., Vicky Conn, R.N., M.N., M.A.; and Barbara Huff

To understand the consumer and family perspectives regarding issues surrounding psychopharmacology, members of the ANA Task Force invited the above family members and consumers to participate in the conference. Margaret Sullivan, co-director of On Our Own, a consumer advocacy group in Baltimore, was invited but was unable to attend. Consequently, this document reflects the perspectives of family members and the respective organizations that they represent, which are identified at the end of this document.

Each participant discussed in different ways a common theme. The theme was that in order to help the families and consumers on the issue of medication management nurses need to be *experts* in understanding the neurobiological disorders, which include the schizophrenias, the affective disorders, obsessive-compulsive disorders, autism, anxiety and panic disorders, pervasive developmental disorders, conduct and attention-deficit hyperactivity disorders, among others. Next, it is assumed that advanced psychiatric nurses have knowledge about efficacious psychopharmacological treatments, which includes understanding side and toxic effects, potential drug interactions, necessary medication monitoring, and management regimes. Many surveys of families indicate that they want to be educated about the medication that their mentally ill family member receives (Hatfield 1981; Hatfield 1990; Francell, Conn, and Gray 1988; McElroy 1987; Spaniol et al. 1984).

In addition, it was recommended that nurses consider a host of other factors that relate to implementing the treatment plan, which includes the phenomenology of the illness. Professionals need to listen to what the family says about the impact of the illness on them, in order to understand the family perspective. They should also listen to the family's description about what medication and other treatments have helped and hindered the patient's progress in the past. Written documentation of medication taken and the responses of the patient need to be developed as critical

components of long-term treatment planning which is maintained and kept by consumers and/or families. These records can be given to new professionals as treatment plans are developed or changed. Assistance from nurses with the development of such written medication formats would be helpful.

Concern was also expressed about taking action when a physician orders medication that seriously exceeds the recommended dosage for a patient. A discussion about overmedication among patients in both adult and child psychiatric hospitals occurred with recommendations that advocacy for these persons needs to occur among nurses when they are confronted with these circumstances. Attention also needs to be directed in instances where, when indicated, there is a failure to provide medication to consumers. This is likely to occur among some staff, in child psychiatric settings, who do not choose to medicate youth, even though evidence exists that such therapy may help the youngster progress (Karahasan 1988; Peschel et al. 1992; Howe and Howe 1992). Specific advocacy strategies for addressing these problems need to be developed in schools of nursing.

Professionals need to inform the family about the care their relative receives in ways that are commensurate with other areas of practice, such as the pediatric unit. On pediatric wards professionals are sensitive to the fact that parents and other family members have a legitimate right to know how the ill person is responding to treatment and that the parents should be considered allies with professionals. Nurses do not hide behind the notion of confidentiality to control and/or to distance themselves from the legitimate and caring concern of other family members, who are also affected by the catastrophic illness of their relative. Staff in other medical subspecialties are governed by the same rules of confidentiality required by mental health professionals; yet most manage to help families by responding helpfully at these times of crisis. These caring staff responses to families in pediatric hospitals and intensive care units could be role models for many psychiatric staff to emulate.

Other recommendations proposed by the presenters were:

1. to individualize the care and avoid standardized behavioral management approaches;
2. to provide active treatment, not custodial care;
3. to develop special programs for those persons who suffer simultaneously from substance abuse and "mental" illness;
4. to know the difference between sociologically based illnesses, such as those associated with poverty, stress, and abuse, and those that are biologically based, since different treatment approaches are required;
5. to practice the highest standards of nursing practice, including responding when legal and ethical aspects of care are compromised.

The preliminary report (this volume) from faculty respondents to the Psychopharmacology Task Force Educational Survey indicated several areas in their curriculum regarding psychopharmacology that raise important questions concerning the inclusion of information on neuroscience, genetics, the biology of psychiatric illnesses, and clinical psychopharmacology, among others. For example, a substantial hereditary component in schizophrenia is one of the two or three best established facts in psychiatry (Bailey and Pillard 1993; Gottesman 1991; Kallmann 1946; Plomin and Daniels 1987) and deserves to be addressed in programs preparing psychiatric nurses.

In summary, efforts to implement in every school of nursing systematic content on the neurobiological aspects of the psychiatric disorders and treatment approaches that have scientific validity from controlled, prospective studies need to occur. A biopsychosocial model that consistently incorporates the "biological" with psychosocial components is again recommended (NIMH 1990). Comprehensive knowledge about psychopharmacology, and medication management and monitoring needs to be reflected in depth in the curriculum as do assessment skills. A core competency that needs to run throughout the curriculum is competency in collaboration with patients, their family care givers, and other mental illness professionals. Persons with these previously mentioned neurobiologically based brain disorders have real illnesses that always require professionals to remember that fact, to reassess their medical status, and to incorporate these important biological factors into their "psychosocial" interventions with patients and their collaborations with families. Attention to such neuroscientific findings would revolutionize how the curriculum in

schools of nursing is taught, change how patients are regarded, and create new directions for working with families as allies with professionals (Hatfield 1990; Marsh 1992; McElroy 1988; Peschel et al. 1992; Moller and Wer 1989).

Members of the ANA Task Force are to be commended for initiating this important national survey among schools of nursing for the purpose of learning more about what and how psychopharmacology is being taught to nurses.

Affiliations of Panel Members

Barbara Huff
The Federation of Families for Children's Mental Health
1021 Prince Street
Alexandria, VA 22314

Vicky Conn, M.A., R.N., M.N.
Chair, Curriculum and Training Committee
The National Alliance for the Mentally Ill
2101 Wilson Boulevard, Suite 302
Arlington, VA 22201

Evelyn McElroy, Ph.D., R.N.
School of Nursing
University of Maryland at Baltimore
655 W. Lombard Street
Baltimore, MD 21201

References

Bailey, J.M., and Pillard, R.C. 1993. Reply to "A genetic study of male sexual orientation." *Archives of General Psychiatry* 50:240-241.

National Institutes of Mental Health, *Clinical training in serious mental illness.* Harriet P. Lefley, ed. 75-96. Washington, DC: U.S. Government Printing Office.

Francell, C., Conn, V., and Gray, D.P. 1988. Families' perceptions of burden of care for chronic mentally ill relatives. *Hospital and Community Psychiatry* 39:1296-1300.

Gottesman, I. 1991. *Schizophrenia genesis: The origins of madness.* New York: WH Freeman.

Hatfield, A.B. 1981. Coping effectiveness in families of the mentally ill: An exploratory study. *Journal of Psychiatric Treatment and Evaluation* 3:11-19.

Hatfield, A.B. 1982. Therapists and families: Worlds apart, *Hospital and Community Psychiatry* 33, 513.

Hatfield, A.B. 1990. *Family education in mental illness.* New York: Guilford Press.

Kallmann, F.J. 1946: The genetic theory of schizophrenia. *American Journal of Psychiatry* 103:309-322.

Karahasan, A. 1988. Common mental illnesses: Symptoms and treatment. In *Children and adolescents with mental illness: A parents' guide,* E. McElroy, ed. 1-31. Kensington, MD: Woodbine House.

Marsh, D. 1992. *Families and mental illness: New directions,* New York: Praeger Publishers.

McElroy, E. 1987. The beat of a different drummer. In *Families of the mentally ill: Coping and adaptation,* A. Hatfield and H. Lefley, eds. New York: Guilford Press, 225-243.

Moller, M., and Wer, J. 1989. Simultaneous patient/family education regarding schizophrenia: The Nebraska model. *Archives of Psychiatric Nurses* III, 6:332-337.

Peschel, E., Peschel, R. Howe, C.W., and Howe, J. 1992. Neurobiological disorders in children and adolescents. *New Directions for Mental Health Services.* 54.

Plomin, R., and Daniels, D. 1987. Why are children in the same family so different from each other? *Brain Science* 10:1-16.

Spaniol, L., Jung, H., Zipple, A.M., and Fitzgerald, S. 1984. *Families as a central resource in the rehabilitation of the severely psychiatrically disabled: Report of a national survey.* Boston: Boston University Center for Rehabilitation Research and Training in Mental Health.

Psychiatric Mental Health Nursing Psychopharmacology Project

SUMMARY REPORT

AMERICAN NURSES ASSOCIATION

American Nurses Association
Task Force on Psychopharmacology
1992-1994

Michele T. Laraia, M.S.N., R.N., Task Force Chair

Linda S. Beeber, Ph.D., R.N.

Gloria B. Callwood, Ph.D., R.N.

Susan Caverly, M.A., R.N.

Jeanne Anne Clement, Ed.D., R.N.

Faye Gary, Ed.D., R.N.

Norman L. Keltner, Ed.D., R.N.

Mary Ann Nihart, M.A., R.N.

Lawrence Scahill, M.S.N., M.P.H., R.N.

Susan Simmons-Alling, M.S.N., R.N.

Sarah R. Stanley, M.S., R.N., C.N.A., C.S.

Sandra Talley, M.N., R.N., A.N.P.

This project was completed with support from the Center for Mental Health Services (formerly NIMH), Division of Clinical Training Branch. Special thanks to project consultants:

Carol Bush, Ph.D., R.N.

Karen Soeken, Ph.D.

Winifred Carson, Esq.

Published by American Nurses Publishing
600 Maryland Avenue, SW
Suite 100 West
Washington, DC 20024-2571

PMH-13(S) 10M 5/94

Table of Contents

Foreword

This publication is a brief summary taken from the report of the work of the American Nurses Association Psychopharmacology Task Force. It includes the Task Force document: Psychopharmacology Guidelines for Psychiatric Mental Health Nurses.

Contact ANA for a copy of the full task force report on the psychopharmacology project.

In recent decades, the National Institute of Mental Health (NIMH) has supported the education and training of health care providers for the chronically mentally ill and their families. Psychiatric mental health nurses, from their biopsychosocial perspective, bring to the psychopharmacologic care of patients and families opportunities for medication teaching, administration, management, therapeutic maintenance, integration with the spectrum of interventions, and interdisciplinary collaboration with other health care providers. These established nursing functions are within the scope of psychiatric mental health nursing practice and are ones that are positively received by both patients and families.

The scientific advances of the past decade are changing the understanding of the human brain, mental illness, and biochemical treatments of mental disorders. Psychiatric nurses must continuously integrate the neurosciences, particularly psychopharmacology, into nursing practice to ensure safe and effective care of people with mental illness and the advancement of the specialty. To facilitate this ongoing process, the American Nurses Association (ANA) and NIMH funded the *Psychiatric Mental Health Nursing Psychopharmacology Project* in 1992.

Introduction

Michele T. Laraia, M.S.N., R.N.
Sarah R. Stanley, M.S., R.N., C.N.A., C.S.

he use of psychopharmacologic

gents to treat mental illness

as revolutionized the manner

which consumers of mental

ealth services and the mental

ealth professions view etiology,

agnosis, treatment, and cost

mental health care in this

untry. Consequently, there

we been a number of

portant changes in the

ental health field in recent

cades.

For example, the national research agenda in mental health has been altered to promote evolving information and technologies. Mental health advocacy groups have been formed and have become a valuable voice in defining the mental health agenda today. The role of psychopharmacologic agents, both as research "probes"—unraveling the etiologies of mental illness and the bases of human behavior—and as powerful treatment tools, which may eventually reach every patient with psychiatric symptoms at one time or another, have expanded to levels of unprecedented sophistication in just a few brief decades.

In response, the roles of the four core mental health professions: psychiatric nursing, psychiatry, psychology, and social work, are being examined and refined to meet these new challenges. The multifaceted nature of mental illness and the complex care required for persons with mental illness necessitate the advantages afforded by the combined efforts of each discipline in the field of mental health care. Interdisciplinary collaboration will continue to provide the vehicle necessary for the most effective treatment and research efforts for the millions of persons suffering from these devastating illnesses.

In this, the "Decade of the Brain," the concerted attempts to apply neuroscientific principals to the understanding and treatment of mental illness will only become more pronounced. These efforts will result in new approaches to the diagnoses and treatments of mental illness, as well as elicit new hope for those who are consumers of mental health services.

To serve the needs of the many people with mental illness, and to remain effective health care providers and capable colleagues within the interdisciplinary mental health care arena, it is imperative that psychiatric mental health nurses remain actively involved in these rapid advances in the mental health field. As we reach the midpoint of the '90s, the specialty of psychiatric mental health nursing is at a critical juncture to move forward in the direction of future education, treatment, and research in the field of mental health.

Meeting these challenges assures that patients and families will have access to the expert skills and resources of one of the largest groups of mental health care professionals, psychiatric nurses. At no other point in modern time has there been such a clearly defined window of opportunity for the specialty of psychiatric mental health nursing to advance in the science and art of mental health care.

Psychiatric nurses are among the primary health care professionals working on a daily basis with the long-term management of psychiatric patients on the continuum of prevention, diagnosis, treatment, maintenance, and rehabilitation. Given the present array of treatment options, this nursing management includes considerable attention to psychopharmacological agents, concurrent health problems, and complex interactions between behavioral, emotional, physiological, and psychopharmacologic events.

Psychiatric mental health nurses are unique in that their training and experience enable them to assess the biological as well as psychosocial needs of patients. Psychiatric mental health nurses will continue to refine and demonstrate their long-standing role in the mental health field, particularly regarding psychopharmacologic treatment and the education of patients and their families about psychopharmacologic agents.

The American Nurses Association Psychopharmacology Project was conceptualized to evaluate and advance the scope of psychiatric nursing practice with respect to psychopharmacology and related neurosciences for both the psychiatric nurse clinician with an undergraduate nursing degree and the advanced-practice psychiatric clinical nurse specialist with a graduate degree in psychiatric mental health nursing.

Purpose

The purpose of the ANA Psychopharmacology Project was to improve psychopharmacologic treatment and educational services to persons with serious mental illness and their families by improving the expertise of psychiatric nurses to deliver those services.

Objectives

The specific objectives of the Psychopharmacology Project were:

1. to determine how well nursing education prepares nurses for practice in the treatment of the mentally ill with respect to psychopharmacology and related neurosciences;

2. to determine how well nursing as a profession facilitates the continued expertise of psychiatric nurses with respect to the evolving content of psychopharmacology and related neurosciences;

3. to define the psychopharmacologic and neuroscientific knowledge base necessary in contemporary psychiatric nursing practice; and,

4. to develop guidelines for psychiatric mental health nurses in psychopharmacology and related neurosciences for the treatment of persons with mental illness.

Methods

The Psychopharmacology Project used several methods to achieve these objectives:

The ANA appointed a representative group of psychiatric mental health nurses to the Psychopharmacology Task Force. These 12 psychiatric mental health nurse specialists, whose names are listed at the beginning of this book, are recognized for their interest, expertise, and leadership in psychopharmacologic treatment, education, and research. Task force members assumed primary responsibility for meeting the objectives of the Psychopharmacology Project. The task force membership reflects a diversity in gender, race, age, affiliation, educational background, state nurses associations (SNAs), and specialty organizations.

Five *content* areas were defined by the task force as guides for organizing the information gathered during the Psychopharmacology Project. These content areas were selected from literature reviews as well as the collective expertise of the task force members regarding the scope of practice of psychiatric mental health nurses working with psychopharmacologic agents.

The members met to plan the implementation of the Psychopharmacology Project and to identify relevant issues in psychopharmacology in nursing practice. This long list of issues was then organized into the following five content areas:

- Neurosciences
- Psychopharmacology
- Assessment
- Clinical Management
- Legal/Ethical Issues

The nursing *environment* is defined as the contribution of the nursing profession regarding education, publications, presentations, and practice in psychiatric nursing. It is from this environment that psychiatric mental health nurses learn about and remain current in psychopharmacology. The environment was evaluated in several ways:

Education: An *educational survey* was developed and sent to every nursing program accredited by the National League for Nursing (NLN). Schools of nursing were asked to provide detailed information about their curricula on psychiatric nursing, psychopharmacology, and related neurosciences.

Publications and Presentations: The following resources were reviewed for content in psychopharmacology and related neurosciences:

- psychiatric nursing textbooks,
- psychiatric nursing journals,
- computer resources and videos, and
- psychiatric nursing conference programs.

Practice: A *National Psychopharmacology Working Conference* of psychiatric mental health nurses recommended by their SNAs was convened. The purpose of this conference was to evaluate nurses' use of psychopharmacological interventions in their work with mentally ill patients and families, and the psychopharmacologic and neuroscientific content that psychiatric nurses in practice need to know.

Consumers of mental health services were invited to participate in the Psychopharmacology Project. Representatives of the National Alliance for the Mentally Ill and The Federation of Families for Children's Mental Health attended the National Psychopharmacology Working Conference and shared their perspectives to the conference participants.

The Psychopharmacology Task Force synthesized the information gained from the Psychopharmacology Project methods described above and developed the *Psychopharmacology Guidelines for Psychiatric Mental Health Nurses*. This document presents guidelines for psychiatric mental health nurses to work at optimal proficiency with patients who receive psychopharmacologic agents as treatments for mental illness. The guidelines are presented in full in Part II, Section 5.

American Nurses Association

Psychopharmacology Guidelines for Psychiatric Mental Health Nurses

The contemporary practice of psychiatric mental health nursing is based on the integration and application of information from the biological, behavioral, social, and neurosciences. Each of these fields is expanding rapidly, requiring ongoing education to ensure incorporation of new findings into psychiatric mental health nursing practice.

This document describes the knowledge base psychiatric mental health nurses need in relation to one aspect of practice—psychopharmacology. It is intended to inform and guide psychiatric mental health nursing education, practice, and research in this area. Thus, this document should not be considered part of any state's nurse practice act, or viewed as a requirement for licensure, or construed as a legal standard by which to judge psychiatric nursing practice.

It is anticipated that these guidelines will regularly be evaluated and updated and that psychiatric mental health nurses will demonstrate expanding expertise in psychopharmacology based on the state of the science, education, experience, practice setting, patient needs, and professional goals.

I. Neurosciences

Commensurate with level of practice, the psychiatric mental health nurse integrates current knowledge from the neurosciences to understand etiological models, diagnostic issues, and treatment strategies for psychiatric illness.

Objectives

The psychiatric mental health nurse can:

- describe basic central nervous system structures and functions implicated in mental illness, such as the cerebrum, diencephalon, brain stem, basal ganglia, limbic system, and extrapyramidal motor system.
- describe basic mechanisms of neurotransmission at the synapse, such as neurochemical metabolism, role of the pre- and post-synaptic membranes, re-uptake, receptor binding, and auto-regulation.
- describe the general functions of the major neurochemicals implicated in mental illness, such as serotonin, norepinephrine, dopamine, acetylcholine, GABA, and the peptides.

- describe the basic structure and function of the endocrine system, particularly as it is affected by the various hypothalamic-pituitary endocrine axes.
- identify the neurotransmitter system implicated in side-effect profiles of psychopharmacologic agents, such as blockade of cholinergic receptors (blurred vision, dry mouth, memory dysfunction), histaminic receptors (sedation, weight gain, hypotension), and adrenergic receptors (dizziness, postural hypotension, tachycardia).
- discuss the relevance of current biological hypotheses underlying major mental illnesses and the use of psychopharmacologic agents.
- demonstrate a familiarity with the increased lifetime risk of mental illness—for people who have a mentally ill first-degree (biological) relative—compared to the general population, based on genetic, epidemiologic, family, adoption, and twin research.
- describe normal sleep stages and identify circadian rhythm disturbances, such as decreased REM latency and phase shift disturbances as evidenced in psychiatric disorders.
- demonstrate familiarity with recent research findings from neuro-imaging techniques such as CT (computerized tomography), MRI (magnetic resonance imagining), PET (positron-emission tomography), and SPECT (single photon emission computerized tomography) as well as the psychiatric uses of these techniques.
- discuss the purposes and limitations of current biological tests used in the diagnosis and monitoring of mental illness.

II. Psychopharmacology

The psychiatric mental health nurse involved in the care of patients who have been prescribed psychopharmacologic agents demonstrates knowledge of psychopharmacologic principles—including pharmacokinetics, pharmacodynamics, drug classification, intended and unintended effects, and related nursing implications.

Objectives
The psychiatric mental health nurse can:

- describe psychopharmacologic agents based on the similarities and differences among drugs of the same and different classes.

- discuss the actions of psychopharmacologic agents that range from global human behavioral responses to those at a cellular level, such as the actions of lithium from mood stabilization to glomerular effects.
- differentiate the psychiatric symptoms targeted for psychopharmacologic intervention from medication side effects and toxicities, and the appropriate interventions to minimize each.
- apply basic principles of pharmacokinetics and pharmacodynamics, such as half-life, steady state, absorption, and metabolism, in general and as they relate to age, gender, race/ethnicity, and organ system function.
- identify the appropriate use of psychotherapeutic agents related to the psychiatric needs of special populations.
- involve patients and their families and significant others in the design and implementation of the medication treatment plan, taking into account patient readiness, knowledge, environment, beliefs and preferences, and lifestyle.
- identify factors that may prevent the active collaboration of patients with medication regimens, and strategies to minimize these risks.
- describe nonpsychopharmacologic interventions for target symptoms that are not responsive to psychopharmacologic interventions, psychiatric symptoms unlikely to respond to drug treatments, and drug side effects that are not treated with drugs.
- discuss the use of standardized rating scales for measuring symptom severity and clinical response to psychopharmacologic treatment, such as changes in target symptoms of illness and medication side effects.
- demonstrate the knowledge necessary to develop psychopharmacologic education and treatment plans based on current neurobiological concepts and the patient's lifestyle and recovery environment.

III. Clinical Management

The psychiatric mental health nurse applies principles from the neurosciences and psychopharmacology to provide safe and effective management of patients being treated with psychopharmacologic agents. Clinical management includes assessment, diagnosis, and treatment considerations.

A. ASSESSMENT

The psychiatric mental health nurse has the knowledge, skills, and ability to conduct and interpret patient assessments in relation to psychopharmacologic agents. Assessments include physical, neuropsychiatric, psychosocial, and psychopharmacologic parameters.

1. Physical Assessment

Objectives
   The psychiatric mental health nurse can:

- collect health data related to past and present health problems and concurrent treatments for other psychiatric or medical problems the patient may have.
- collect health data related to current and past drug use (prescribed, over-the-counter, and illicit), current and past substance use (caffeine, nicotine, alcohol), and related health practices.
- conduct and/or interpret findings from a physical examination and laboratory studies to obtain information about pertinent organ system functioning.
- evaluate laboratory results that reflect drug effects on organ systems, drug blood levels and toxicities, and concurrent medical problems that may mimic or exacerbate psychiatric symptoms or drug effects.
- assess a baseline and ongoing status of motor activity and sleep patterns, appetite, dietary practices and preferences, and functional status.

2. Neuropsychiatric Assessment

Objectives
   The psychiatric mental health nurse can:

- conduct and/or interpret findings from a basic neuropsychiatric exam including gross cranial and peripheral nerve function; gait; muscle strength, function and range of motion; and mental status.
- identify chief neuropsychiatric complaints, presenting symptoms, and goals for psychopharmacologic interventions.
- make appropriate use of available informants and records to augment self-reports of neuropsychiatric assessment and premorbid patterns.
- demonstrate appropriate use of standardized rating scales to document mental status, drug effects on the core psychiatric symptomatology, and side effects such as those occurring in the extrapyramidal system.

3. Psychosocial Assessment

Objectives
   The psychiatric mental health nurse can:

- utilize demographic and personal information for the development of a patient-centered medication treatment plan considering the patient's ethnic/cultural background, developmental stage, cognitive ability, educational level, reading level and comprehension, socioeconomic status, and capacity to ask questions and seek answers.
- assess the effects of psychopharmacologic interventions on the patient's quality of life including the impact on interpersonal relationships, appearance, work and leisure functioning, diet, sleep, sexual performance, family planning, functional status, financial status, self-esteem, and perception of stigma associated with medication intervention.
- identify actual and potential sources of support for the patient such as significant others; household and family members; friendships and informal relationships; work relationships; and affiliations with community, social, and religious organizations.
- identify actual and potential barriers to treatment within the patient and the environment, such as impaired functional status, cultural/ethnic/religious beliefs and practices, absence of a support system, limited cognitive abilities, stressors, financial hardships, deficient coping skills, impaired capacity to collaborate with treatment, limited transportation, and patient and family perceptions of illness and medication treatment.

4. Psychopharmacological Assessment

Objectives
   The psychiatric mental health nurse can:

- identify patient-related variables pertinent to the risk/benefit assessment of psychopharmacologic treatment such as demographic (age, gender, ethnicity/race); physical (organ system function, concurrent illnesses); treatment (concurrent treatments); and personal (past history, self-care practices, goals for treatment, ability to pay, and quality of life) characteristics.
- identify drug-related variables important in the risk/benefit assessment of psychopharmacologic agents, such as safety and efficacy, advantages and disadvan-

tages compared to other drugs in the same class, therapeutic range, side effect profile, toxicities, contraindications, potential interactions with other drugs or diet, polypharmacy considerations, safety in overdose, availability of information on long-term side effects, and cost.

- evaluate the appropriateness and least restrictive nature of psychopharmacologic interventions for each patient.
- assess the ability and willingness of the patient and significant others to give informed consent for treatment with psychopharmacologic agents.
- utilize standardized behavioral rating scales to assess and monitor drug effects and changes in target symptoms.

B. DIAGNOSIS

The psychiatric mental health nurse has the knowledge, skills, and ability to utilize appropriate nursing, psychiatric, and medical diagnostic classification systems to guide psychopharmacologic management of patients with mental illness.

Objectives
The psychiatric mental health nurse can:

- utilize standardized diagnostic systems as appropriate for making nursing (North American Nursing Diagnostic Association-NANDA or other nursing systems) and psychiatric (*Diagnostic and Statistical Manual—DSM*) diagnoses, and interpreting medical diagnoses (*International Classification of Diseases—ICD*).
- elicit information from the patient—and other appropriate informants or records—that is relevant to the diagnostic process.
- make nursing diagnostic judgments that include information about but are not limited to the psychiatric diagnosis, symptoms targeted for psychopharmacologic intervention, medical diagnoses, physical symptoms, coping responses, functional status, developmental level, learning capabilities, and the patient's quality of life and preferences.
- use these diagnostic judgments as the basis for setting treatment priorities and selecting and assessing nursing interventions, including management of psychopharmacologic agents.

- communicate and integrate diagnostic impressions with other members of the health care team. This can include representatives of managed care enterprises.

C. TREATMENT

The psychiatric mental health nurse takes an active role in the treatment of patients with mental illness and integrates prescribed psychopharmacologic interventions into a cohesive, multidimensional plan of care.

1. Initiation

Objectives
The psychiatric mental health nurse can:

- use information obtained during the nursing assessment to develop a medication treatment plan that considers target symptoms, side effects, concurrent treatments and health status, requirements of specific drugs, dietary and activity considerations, and patient-related variables.
- demonstrate an understanding of pharmacokinetic and pharmacodynamic principles that underlie safe and effective psychopharmacologic management, such as how dosing and tapering schedules are adjusted, and how patient-related variables are integrated.
- relate the length of time it may take a drug to have a therapeutic effect, the time it takes for expected side effects to occur and remit, early signs of unexpected or adverse events, and nursing interventions to reduce side effects and facilitate therapeutic response.
- apply principles of health education, nursing ethics, and legal parameters in informing patients about medication treatments, risks/benefits, concurrent and alternative treatments, and informed consent.
- apply least restrictive principles and advance directives to avoid the overuse or under-use of medications as chemical restraints, and to anticipate safety needs, such as potential for harm to self or others, suicidality, aggression, assaultiveness, and violence.

2. Stabilization

Objectives
The psychiatric mental health nurse can:

- monitor target symptoms, acute medication effects, and functional status throughout the course of treatment.
- utilize information obtained from therapeutic drug monitoring, laboratory values, standardized rating scales, and patient and family reports to monitor progress.
- recognize indications for modifying dosing schedules and describe alternative medication strategies as needed.

3. Maintenance

Objectives
The psychiatric mental health nurse can:

- develop a plan of care in collaboration with the patient, family, and other care providers as appropriate, that includes monitoring outcomes such as efficacy of treatment, changes in target symptoms, emergence of long-term side effects, laboratory values and physical findings relevant to specific medications, and occurrence of destabilizing stressors.
- identify possible barriers to maintenance care, such as issues regarding transportation, finances, birth control, child care, support system, relocation, cultural/ethnic differences, therapeutic relationship, and psychosocial stressors, as well as the patient's understanding of symptom reduction, symptom exacerbation, and side effects.
- facilitate the patient's transition from one treatment setting to another, such as from the hospital to the community, from one care provider to another, and from one treatment to another.
- develop a patient-education program for relapse prevention that may include self-monitoring techniques and teaching tools such as medication cards, handouts, diaries, bibliographies, and other materials to enhance ongoing education of patients, families, and significant others.
- enhance health promotion with restoration techniques that can be individualized for the patient and integrated with medication treatments, such as diet; exercise; leisure activities; and community, social, and religious affiliations.
- assist the patient, family, and significant others to establish advance directives regarding emergency interventions, including the use of psychopharmacologic agents.

4. Discontinuation and Follow-Up

Objectives
The psychiatric mental health nurse can:

- relate current recommended practices regarding psychopharmacologic maintenance requirements and duration of treatment for specific psychiatric disorders.
- discuss issues related to discontinuation of medication, including tapering schedules, and potential sequelae such as withdrawal, dependence, rebound effects, and return of symptoms of illness.
- develop with the patient, family, and significant others a plan for self-care in a post-medication phase that considers assessments of quality of life, predisposing stressors, re-emergence of symptoms, appropriate use of support systems, and contact sources for potential re-evaluation of treatment status.
- assess the patient before, during, and after the course of treatment, clearly differentiating between changes in the patient as a result of illness effects, drug effects, premorbid personality characteristics, effects of aging, and effects of the environment.

IV. Recommendations

These *Guidelines* are designed to be used as a tool for psychiatric mental health nurses to determine their knowledge and skill in psychopharmacology, and to design a plan for their continued growth in this field. The *Guidelines* can also be used as the basis for the development of curricula and continuing education programs for psychiatric mental health nurses in psychopharmacology. New information in this field should be added to the *Guidelines* on a regular basis.

As a set of guidelines, this document should not be used in legal proceedings or as an evaluation of nurses' competence in this field by institutions or state or federal agencies.

Summary and Recommendations

This summary of the findings from the Psychopharmacology Project reflects two years of work and the effort of many individuals. Hopefully, the recommendations will provide a basis for the increased integration of psychopharmacology content into the formal and informal educational programs of nurses, as well as the fuller application of this information in quality nursing care provided to persons with mental illness and their families.

One initiative of the Psychopharmacology Project was an evaluation of the psychiatric mental health nursing environment related to psychopharmacology. This environmental review included: education, publications (textbooks, journals, computer programs, and videos), and conferences. This review proved useful in documenting what is currently provided within the specialty for psychiatric mental health nurses related to psychopharmacology.

In addition, the practice setting environment for psychiatric mental health nurses was reviewed. A National Conference on Competencies in Psychopharmacology for Psychiatric Nurses provided a thorough review of what psychiatric mental health nurses need in the practice setting, related to psychopharmacology and related neuroscience, as articulated by leaders in the field. From the perspective of both clinicians and educators across the country, there is a great and immediate need for information and guidelines by which nurses can pursue ongoing knowledge in the fields of biological psychiatry and psychopharmacology.

The national conference included several people representing consumer advocacy groups for persons with mental illness. Not surprisingly, consumer groups are also challenging mental health professionals to reconsider exclusively psychodynamic explanations of mental illness. This is in light of recent developments in the neurosciences, particularly those involving genetics, the results of neuro-imaging techniques, and the effects of psychopharmacologic agents. These groups believe that the individuals and families they represent have long felt blamed for causing mental illness in their family members.

To ensure that psychiatric mental health nurses are prepared to assimilate and communicate the explosion of critical scientific information in this field, it is essential that a number of changes be made. A rapid step forward in almost all of the areas reviewed is recommended so that psychiatric mental health nurses can continue to turn to their specialty for the information necessary to care for psychiatric patients, teach psychiatric mental health nursing, and conduct research in the specialty.

The number of nurses entering graduate programs in psychiatric nursing has declined over the past two decades. In addition, less than 20 percent of master's-prepared nurses are under 35 years of age (NIMH 1990). Younger nurses are not joining the ranks of psychiatric nursing. The loss of federal funding for graduate education in nursing has played a major role in this decline.

To garner support and attract new students to psychiatric mental health nursing and graduate study in the field, both undergraduate and graduate curricula must keep pace with the developments in the field of mental health, including the neurosciences and psychopharmacology. Failure to do so carries the risk of continuing the decline in the number of psychiatric mental health nurses prepared to practice in this country at a time when the need for mental health professionals has never been greater.

Specifically, undergraduate- and graduate-level nursing programs must include comprehensive and current information about the neurosciences and psychopharmacology as they relate to mental illness. Undergraduate nursing programs should provide a solid foundation in neuroscience and psychopharmacology, while graduate programs in psychiatric mental health nursing should require advanced learning, clinical application, and research inquiry in these essential fields.

As more is learned about the genetic, developmental, and environmental determinants of mental illness, treatment is likely to become increasingly multimodal and multidisciplinary (Institute of Medicine 1989). Therefore, psychiatric nurse clinicians and specialists will need education that extends beyond the traditional modalities of individual, family, and group psychotherapy (Krauss 1993).

Given the proliferation of physiological tests, psychopharmacologic agents, and other somatic treatments, added educational effort in this area is essential. Closely related clinical skills, such as physical assessment, medication management, and the use of valid and reliable methods of monitoring drug response are equally important. Mastering this content and articulating the roles of psychiatric mental health nurses in these rapidly expanding areas will offer exciting career opportunities for nurses entering the specialty, while access to mental health services and the quality of care provided patients with psychiatric illness will be improved.

While psychiatric nursing publications have shown an increased focus on psychopharmacology and the neurosciences over the past few years, they need additional content to provide nurses with current, comprehensive information in these rapidly changing fields. These publications have a wide readership and can make an important contribution to continuing education in this area, but it is not clear at present whether editors and authors view the fields of neurosciences, including psychopharmacology, as essential areas of psychiatric nursing practice.

Furthermore, in this age of expanding automated services, psychiatric mental health nurses must be better able to access information in an automated format. Changes need to be made to facilitate nurses' computerized searches of databases related to journal articles and computer-assisted learning programs. These technologies must be utilized in today's rapidly changing health care environment so the profession can keep up with critical information necessary to provide excellence in patient care, based upon the integration of new theories, interventions, and research findings.

Psychiatric nursing conferences are a resource to the field in their presentation and dissemination of information about psychopharmacology and related neurosciences to nurse clinicians and specialists. The number of pre-conference workshops and conference presentations in these areas has been increasing over the past few years and almost every major psychiatric nursing conference program now includes these topics, indicating the high nurse-consumer demand for this information. Funding for conferences offering this information, as well as scholarships for those attending these conferences, should be made available to continue to support this important learning resource in this age of dwindling health care training and education funds.

The *Psychopharmacology Guidelines for Psychiatric Mental Health Nurses* is the definitive outcome of the Psychopharmacology Project. The *Guidelines* should be disseminated to all psychiatric mental health nurses, every institution in which nurses are educated, and each practice setting where patients receive care. They should be used as guides to direct changes in the way psychiatric mental health nurses view their roles in the care of the mentally ill; advocacy for mentally ill patients and their families; education of psychiatric nurses; research in evolving areas of practice; and interdisciplinary collaboration with other professionals in the health care field.

The ANA Task Force on Psychopharmacology therefore proposes that NIMH and ANA call for a national initiative to support the knowledge base and role of psychiatric mental health nurses in the administration, health education, and therapeutic maintenance of patients receiving psychopharmacologic medications. The future should include the refinement of levels of psychopharmacology practice by psychiatric mental health nurses, including the appropriate credentialing of psychiatric mental health nurses in psychopharmacology.

In addition, training grants for nursing programs—particularly at the graduate level—that demonstrate contemporary course work in psychopharmacology and related neurosciences should be made available to attract promising students to the specialty and to support them. Grant money for fellowships for pre-doctoral nurses in these fields will greatly enhance the treatment and research components of the specialty of psychiatric mental health nursing. Post-doctoral fellowships should be offered to nurses working in these fields at salaries commensurate with their experience and education.

Because of the rapid and comprehensive changes, related to psychopharmacology, needed in the nursing environment, continuing education programs in the neurosciences and psychopharmacology should be supported, continuously updated, and made available to all psychiatric mental health nurses.

Equally important, legislation and regulations should allow patients access to psychiatric mental health nurses as primary mental health care providers; allow reimbursement for the services they provide; and reduce unnecessary federal and state restrictions on their practice. Finally, at every level, government and private agencies should include psychiatric nurses on regulatory and decision-making panels and commissions regarding mental health diagnosis, treatment, and service delivery issues.

This is a time of unprecedented change and opportunity within the health and mental health care fields. The specialty of psychiatric mental health nursing and the profession of nursing as a whole, will be greatly affected by every initiative and strategy that is developed as a result of the findings of the Psychopharmacology Project and the *Psychopharmacology Guidelines for Psychiatric Mental Health Nurses*. Most of all, however, the responsibility for action lies with the individual nurse and with psychiatric mental health nurses as a group to keep abreast of knowledge in their field and apply it on a daily basis in the care of patients with mental illness and their families.

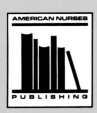

American Nurses Publishing
is the publishing program of
the American Nurses Foundation,
an affiliate organization of the
American Nurses Association.

PMH-13(S) 10M 5/94